W0050852

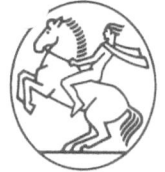

Disorders of Human Communication 7

Edited by G.E.Arnold, F.Winckel, B.D.Wyke
Executive Editor: B.D.Wyke

Margaret Edwards
Disorders
of Articulation

Aspects of Dysarthria
and Verbal Dyspraxia

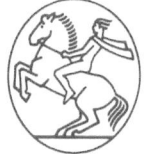

Springer-Verlag Wien New York

Margaret Edwards

Institute of Neurology, University of London, Great Britain

With 18 Figures

Library of Congress Cataloging in Publication Data. Edwards. Margaret. 1924–. Disorders of articulation. (Disorders of human communication ; 7.) Bibliography : p. Includes indexes. 1. Articulation disorders. I. Title. II. Series [DNLM : 1. Speech disorders. 2. Apraxia. 3. Speech – Physiology W1 DI762 v. 7 / WL 340 E26d]. RC424.7.E38. 1984. 616.85′5. 84-5350

ISSN 0173-170X
ISBN-13:978-3-7091-8737-1   e-ISBN-13:978-3-7091-8735-7
DOI: 10.1007/978-3-7091-8735-7

Preface

The title of this book may at first appear to be somewhat restrictive in its use of terminology. However, this is far from the intention of the writer; on the contrary, the following chapters seek to reflect a departure from the traditional segmentally orientated approach to this type of disability. Indeed one reason why the book has been written is the sense of frustration arising out of the largely ineffectual static and structural methodology of remedial work.

Alternative titles could have been Disorders of Speech Production, or Neurogenic Speech Disorders, but neither would have encapsulated the essence of the book.

Much of the recent research in the neurophysiology of motor control and also in the field of neurolinguistics has been concerned with ways in which intention and planning of movement is effected. Such models are still in their infancy, but it seems the potential value of their application to speech is considerable. In the case of verbal dyspraxia, for example, we have long since in rather vague terms described it as a disorder of organization and programming without ever stating exactly what may be disorganized or not properly planned.

This book does not provide the answer for as yet there is insufficient data on which to work so that formulated theories may be tested and further defined. But as we move from speculative guess-work towards established fact so the likelihood grows of providing more positive help for those who suffer these drastic limitations in communication.

This work therefore is not intended to be a comprehensive account of articulatory disorders but is rather a selection of those conditions which best exemplify disorders which appear to be associated with the planning and control functions of the central nervous system.

While the focus is on supraglottic articulatory aspects, it will be readily apparent to the reader that a fragmented account such as the title might imply is unacceptable and that throughout the text there is an endeavour to stress the holistic nature of speech production.

As well as informing, it is hoped that the ensuing chapters will act as a stimulus to those clinicians who have access to such a wealth of information based on clinical experience. Perhaps they will examine their records more closely with the object of either substantiating or refuting the views expressed herein and in turn of generating further work which may help their patients.

London, June 1984   **Margaret Edwards**

Acknowledgements

My first acknowledgement of help received must be to Professor Barry Wyke. Not only has he helped to bring up to date my views on neuroanatomy and neurophysiology but he has also proved to be a ruthless eradicator of split infinitives and inappropriate whimsical punctuation.

Then I should like to thank Dr. John Laver for the generosity he has shown in sharing some of his ideas with me. The frequency of reference to his work is a testimony to their value.

My colleagues in Nottinghamshire have unfailingly alerted me to the arrival of patients whose conditions has been of special interest and I am most grateful for their enthusiasm.

Competing demands of writing and a full time job in a service presently undergoing drastic change have inevitably produced irritability and I should like to thank my mother for her forbearance and understanding when such pressures have been considerable.

Lastly Elizabeth Jennings has without a murmur of protest painstakingly transcribed the frenetic writing into neat and legible type and I am indeed grateful for her support.

With all this help, the blame for shortcomings within the book must be mine alone.

Margaret Edwards

Contents

What Is Meant by Disorders of Articulation? 1

Introductory chapters by tradition attempt to give the reader a preview of the main content of the book. In the present case there is an additional requirement, namely to consider some of the issues which have determined the particular choice of topics described.

The title itself constitutes a considerable terminological challenge, for the term *articulation* raises many questions and while superficially it appears amenable to a straightforward definition, e.g. "in speech the production of individual sounds in connected discourse" (Wood in Travis, 1971), few readers would now find such a definition acceptable partly because of its lack of comprehensiveness, but mainly in the light of more recent developments in the field of phonology.

Crystal (1982) elaborates on some of the difficulties which arise in trying to define different types of language disability. Assisted by Twiston Davies (forthcoming) he embarked on a project, one aim of which was to consider the breadth and limitations of a traditional system of terminology. Beginning with *articulation* in the belief (mistaken as it turned out) that this might be one of the more direct paths in the labyrinthine jungle of definition and nomenclature they soon realized that because of the diversity of interpretation the task was virtually an impossible one and that they would have to abandon any notion of arriving at a circumscribed definition.

Problems of Classification

At the outset therefore it is important to determine the particular aspects of articulation to be described and to establish the conditions to which they relate. A second issue is that of classification, about which there is also some confusion.

Ingram in 1972 offered a classification of speech and language disorders as applied to children which he based on "linguistic and phonetic" criteria (one sees here in the choice of words yet another instance of ambiguity since many would regard phonetics as being a branch of linguistics). However, here it is taken as being intended to differentiate between different levels of language production.

Under the heading *Disorders of articulation* Ingram lists:

specific development delay
structural dysarthria
neurological dysarthria

Structural dysarthria refers to disorders of speech arising from conditions such as clefts of the palate and other craniofacial abnormalities. By designating these *dysarthria* Ingram extends what is traditionally a neurologically associated term. While etymologically this is acceptable since the root *arthroo* means no more than *articulate* the impression is that this classification has not been widely adopted by clinicians who continue to limit the use of dysarthria to those conditions with a neurological connotation.

Whether one accepts this classification or not, the terms used are still inadequate to define the associated speech disorder, mainly because it gives prominence to one particular aspect of what are essentially disorders involving many levels of speech production.

This book is concerned only with neurological dysarthria (Ingram's terms) and in particular with neurophysiological and neurolinguistic aspects of dysfunction.

Two companion volumes in this series (Crystal, 1981; Martin, 1981) have considered the implications of various types of disorder associated with maturational delay and Crystal has underlined the difficulties inherent in trying to classify what is probably a heterogeneous group of disorders. Specific developmental delay is in any case a somewhat diffuse term which at present it is difficult to clarify.

Structural disorders of articulation also constitute a different group of disorders though there may be some common features underlying the three categories listed by Ingram. These will however be described in greater detail in a forthcoming volume in the series.

Historical Aspects

The early history of the diagnosis of articulatory disorder is an interesting one and is well described in Ynez Viole O'Neill's (1980) fascinating account of the history of speech disorder up to 1600.

Early writings link articulatory disorder with cerebral dysfunction, but associated with both is the notion of humoral pathology. Aristotle mentions excess of moisture in the tongue as being a cause of disorder and much later Galen was still propounding the view that children's immature speech as well as their incoordinated movements were due to a plethora of humidity. In older people the reverse applied and the disorder was then thought to be due to dehydration.

Aristotle in the Problemata Vol. XI defined three types of articulatory impairment, *ischnophonos, traylos,* and *psellos.* Ischnophonos is described as the failure to join one syllable to another with normal speed, traylos is the inability to produce certain sounds, while psellos denotes the omission of sounds and syllables. These features are all familiar components of what we now term dysarthria and dyspraxia of speech.

Mercurialis writing in the late 1500s acknowledges Aristotle's and Galen's theses but he also attributes articulatory disorder to damage to the tongue causing lingual paralysis or, in the complete absence of speech, to a disturbance of the brain.

Throughout the descriptions of articulatory disorder there is a recurring reference to drunkeness as an exacerbating factor influencing humidity. This is of interest because of the close link between cerebellar dysfunction and alcoholism. The disorders described might well be forms of cerebellar ataxia. It is therefore possible that Aristotle and Galen attributed to alcohol, what was in fact ataxic dysarthria not necessarily connected with alcoholic poisoning. Similarly the reference to excess humor producing incoordinate movements in children might betoken the same cause.

Moving on to the late 19th century, John Bristowe, a British neurologist, published a series of lectures in the Lancet in which he described speech mechanisms. In relation to articulation he stated:

". . . and the movements of the lips, jaw, tongue and soft palate shall be accurately adjusted for each literal sound and capable of passing from one set of adjustments to another with rapidity and smoothness."

At about the same time the English translation of Kussmaul's *Disturbances of speech* appeared and in this he designated disorders of articulation originating from either organic or psychic disturbance as dysarthria and differentiated between upper and lower motor neurone lesions.

Among French neurologists considerable controversy was being generated concerning the nature of neurological disorders of speech and Broca's delineation of *aphemia* was greeted with sceptism by many of his contemporaries.

Partly because of personal rivalries there is little evidence of any attempt to link up different investigations and in particular the relationships between dysarthria and aphasia do not appear to have been made explicit. Rockey (1980) comments on the considerable confusion and muddle which existed between classification of aphasia and dysarthria and indeed in the light of present conflict one is tempted to think "Twas ever thus".

Grewel in 1957 provided a comprehensive overview of work relating to dysarthria and offered a taxonomy based on a neurological and linguistic model. He refers to Froment's work published between 1924 and 1935 wherein he defines two phases in word production. The first relates to the praxis of the word(s). The second phase Grewel translates as:

"the setting free of as it were conditioned reflexes that constitute the utterance of these different phonemes" (p. 328)

Such a description anticipates to some extent Hebb's later (1949) thesis of motor schema.

Impairment at the second phase would result in dysarthria. The classification of dysarthria adopted by Grewel is a modification of that described by Peacher (1950). This lists 14 different types of dysarthria each of which relates to an anatomic location or to a specific type of neuropathology. To this medical model Grewel adds what he calls a logopaedic dimension by describing particular types associated with certain neurological states, flaccidity, spasticity, ataxia etc.

The paper is important because it heralds the need to regard dysarthria as more than a disorder of articulation. The importance of investigating respiratory, phonatory and prosodic aspects is stressed. At least progress in this respect can be reported since 1957.

In the parallel field of dyspraxia investigation, Hughlings Jackson and Liepmann were the two most frequently quoted names, the former particularly for the promotion of the close association of the Will with dyspraxic disturbance and the latter in relation to his classification of three levels of dyspraxia; ideational, ideomotor and limb kinetic.

Ideational dyspraxia disrupts the ability to carry out plans of action in their normal sequence. Applied to speech, this suggests an impairment in the selection of appropriate sequences of linguistic units.

Ideomotor dyspraxia presents the obverse side of the coin, in that complex actions are retained but individual components may be disrupted.

Limb kinetic dyspraxia Liepmann suggested was characterized by a loss of kinaesthetic memory for movement of specific parts of the body; in speech, the organs of the vocal tract.

In recent years, views on verbal dyspraxia have been dominated by the extensive research carried out throughout the 60s and 70s at the Mayo Clinic. The exclusively "motor" interpretation of dyspraxia put forward by Darley and his colleagues has served to generate strongly opposing views exemplified by workers like Martin (1974) who, while not disputing the existence of symptoms described by the Mayo school, nevertheless regard them as aphasic rather than motor in origin. At the present time there is as yet no satisfactory resolution of the conflicting claims.

Much of the earlier work concentrated on acquired neuropathology and in keeping with general attitudes children were regarded as miniature immature adults.

Muriel Morley in the late 50s was among the first to describe a specific type of articulatory disorder which she called *developmental articulatory dyspraxia*. At that time she was working closely with neurologists and paediatricians at Newcastle upon Tyne and her observations led her to the belief that among a large group of children labelled as having *dyslalia* it was possible to extrapolate a number (12 in this case) whose articulatory defects separated them markedly from the remainder. Her diagnosis again prompted controversy and indeed has continued to do so.

Whereas in the acquired condition dispute centres not on the existence of dyspraxia but more on whether it is a motor disorder or a type of aphasia, in the developmental condition there are those who maintain that no claim can be made for the delineation of such a group and therefore it does not merit a special label.

Relationship of Articulation to Other Levels of Production

One thing which is apparent throughout all the earlier studies of dyspraxia and dysarthria is the concentration on articulatory aspects of the disorder with little more than passing reference to other parameters of speech production. While a recognition of the importance of these other aspects has grown in relation to dysarthria, for dyspraxia this is not the case. Few of the Mayo studies for example have included a systematic investigation of non segmental features in their research.

There are two important factors which need to be accepted. The first is that dysarthria is not pure and simple a disorder of articulation. Related to this is the fact that in any case articulation cannot be regarded as an isolable entity which may be described without reference to other parameters of production. Greene refers to the "inseparable dualism" of phonation and articulation and in this context she also includes resonance.

Accounts of dyspraxia have likewise concentrated on segmental features but there is no reason why programming deficits should be confined to one component of speech production. Why not respiratory, laryngeal, or resonatory dyspraxia? For example, clinical impressions are of a considerable number of children attending cleft palate centres for investigation of unexplained hypernasality of speech. When structural causes like submucous cleft have been ruled out there remains a possibility of disproportion between nasal and oral pharynx. But other possibilities which need to be considered are isolated suprabulbar paresis or dyspraxic impairment which manifests as faulty timing in the coordination of muscular action to effect the operation of the velopharyngeal sphincter.

Dynamic Nature of Articulation

Where then lies the emphasis in this book? Essentially it is in trying to establish the importance of the dynamic nature of speech production. To do this it is necessary to consider these disorders in the context of current neuro-physiological and neurolinguistic theory and the descriptions which follow are based on these. Theories on control of movement have been evolving steadily since 1949 when Hebb first proposed a theory of motor equivalence.

Similarly in the related field of neurolinguistics there has been a growing emphasis on the planning and programming component of speech production. Drawing upon evidence derived from speech errors and from evidence of anticipatory planning of speech as in coarticulation, speech scientists and psychologists have formulated new theories of production.

Lashley's 1951 paper is one of the corner stones of processing theory. In this he propounds his view of language being the result of "predetermined orderly sequences of action". Later in 1965 the Soviet workers Kozhevnikov and Chistovich developed the notion of the syllable as the unit of planning, and of the *syntagma* which they regarded as a string of up to about seven syllables which were preplanned and activated by a rhythm generator within the central nervous system.

Allied to planning theories, ideas were also being put forward about the way in which output of speech is controlled. Laver basing evidence on research of "slips of the tongue" data in 1970 described a model of production which included a monitoring facility. These earlier views have been followed by further development in subsequent papers (e.g. 1977, 1980a).

It is of interest to note the parallel courses being pursued by neuro-physiologists and neurolinguists at the present time. Just as the latter have moved away from the consideration of speech as a series of separated segments so too have the former with regard to movement. The literature now reflects an increasing focus on the synergistic nature of motor activity.

Closely related to coordination and seriation are properties of rhythm and timing and these aspects also assume importance in the descriptions which follow.

As yet, studies which apply these recent developments to speech disorder are sparse and their relevance to principles of remediation have scarcely been considered, save perhaps for some of the work being carried out at Wisconsin which is of compelling interest.

As ways are found in which theories of distributed control, of preplanning and feedback can be applied to remedial techniques, it is to be hoped that as a result, more satisfactory progress will be made in the alleviation of dysarthria and dyspraxia. Hitherto the emphasis on a rather static "tip of the tongue" approach has not proved particularly successful.

It is partly as the result of an endeavour to focus attention on these dynamic aspects of production that an eclectic course of description has been chosen in the following chapters. At no point is there an intention to offer a comprehensive account of neurogenic speech disorders, but rather to select certain facets which serve to illustrate current theories of planning and control.

Regrettably at the present time one is forced through lack of discriminative data to an acceptance of David Crystal's (1982) comments about terminological confusion. In his discussion of this issue he poses several problems which he applies specifically to the definition of articulatory disorder though he is at pains to point out that this particular condition is not alone in being hedged about by anomalies and ambiguities.

Terms of Reference

These problems which are put in question form, serve, through an attempt to answer them, as a suitable framework in which to summarize the way in which parts of this particular book have evolved.

The first question posed by Crystal is:

i) Is articulation disorder an organic or non organic condition?

In this context only organic conditions are described.

Precisely what range of etiological factors are involved?

The current state of neuropathological investigation still leaves many questions unanswered with regard to neurogenic speech disorders. Where known they are described, and where not confirmed, they are discussed speculatively. The focus is on organic aetiology though it is recognized that other factors, e.g. psychogenic, must contribute, but these are not considered in any detail.

Is there any clear correlation with severity of condition?

Generally yes, but not necessarily in a linear dimension. What is not yet established is the effect upon speech production of the relative predominance of different neuropathological features.

ii) Is it a phonetic or a phonological disorder?

Both. To take the case of dysarthria, the presenting disorder may be phonetic but the speaker's attempts to deal with his handicap through compensatory tactics will result in phonological, morphological, syntactic and possibly semantic change.

Where dyspraxia is concerned the notion of duality is favoured, so that both phonetic and phonological correlates may co-occur in varying degrees of dominance. There are also disorders of prosody both phonetic and phonological and frequently syntactic levels are affected as well.

iii) What is the nature of the units within which the distribution of the articulation disability may be defined?

Certainly not within individual segments as this would belie a preplanning function in production. It is probably necessary to define the disability in terms of tone units in order to provide a comprehensive view. Such a unit would allow for examination of many facets relating to any particular type of disorder, that is to say features of stress, pitch, timing, pause, coarticulation, assimilation and so forth.

iv) Is there a single disorder varying in severity or are there subtypes?

In the present context and certainly with regard to dysarthria subtypes have been established. The literature generally acknowledges the plurality of the condition. With regard to dyspraxia the situation is not as clear and is further clouded by controversy about what is meant exactly by the term. The present text give indications of both sub- and superfluent forms which differ in some respects. Again there is also reference to predominantly phonetic as against phonological types. This raises the question: at what point does phonetic dyspraxia become dysarthria and similarly at what point does phonological dyspraxia become an aphasia? And what constitutes the constellation which is termed dyspraxia along this spectrum? These questions can only be answered by evidence from many more *detailed* case studies. Clinically it is probably more fruitful to regard both dyspraxia, dysarthria and dysphasia as being on a continuum with differing prominence of features determining the present system of labelling.

v) Should other phonological notions be brought into the definitions – such as phonological processes?

Yes, if investigation helps to delineate the condition by establishing whether certain rules are operating. But, and at the present time this is only hazarding a guess, it may well be found that these rules operate so inconsistently as to be of little value in determining patterns. Furthermore processes which may be operating are possibly secondary to neurological correlates as for example in disorders of timing.

Finally to establish the terms of the ensuing discussion another relevant question needs to be asked,

What are the other parameters of speech production involved?

Indications are that articulation must be regarded as *only one component* of speech production. Respiration, phonation, resonance are other interrelated components and a full consideration of speech disability must include their contribution to the totality of the disorder.

Neurophysiological Aspects of Speech Production 2

Classical descriptions of articulatory disorders have tended to be much concerned with analysis of error in the final stages of production. The use of terms like "substitution" and "distortion" borrowed from the literature of developmental assessment protocols demonstrates this tendency. Such classification yields very limited information, whereas a type of analysis focussing on dynamic aspects of the articulatory process might prove to be more fruitful. Laver, writing in 1977 about normal speech production states: "The concentration of phonetic interest on articulation has led to the relative neglect by phoneticians of aspects of speech upstream as it were, from the movement of the peripheral speech apparatus" (p. 142). In relation to disorder such a downstream concentration is likely to limit understanding because underlying dysfunction may be insufficiently taken into account and as a consequence, important strategies for remediation overlooked.

This chapter attempts to describe in outline the neurophysiology underlying speech production. Any description of human behaviour which carries a prefix "neuro" is bound to be incomplete because of constraints on investigation, and if the subject under discussion is speech, the difficulties are even greater. It will be apparent from this and the following chapter which discusses neurolinguistic models, that whereas knowledge of many aspects of human function can be inferred from parallel animal studies, such analogies do not extend to the domain of speech and language. Data have therefore had to be gathered and models formulated on evidence provided by malfunctioning brains (e.g. Penfield and Roberts, 1959), and on that provided by speech itself particularly from errors of speech (e.g. Boomer and Laver, 1968; Fromkin, 1973, 1980).

The increasing availability too of sensitive technology offers opportunity for further insight into processes underlying speech, as well as greater accuracy in measurement and description of speech production.

Theories about the neurology of speech are however still besprent with a fair amount of conflicting speculation and the following account for this reason confines itself to more established and therefore less detailed aspects.

Cerebral Dominance

Articulatory structures though bilaterally innervated are probably unilaterally controlled. Evidence from a number of studies (Semmes, 1968; Kimura and Archbold, 1974) indicate that the dominant hemisphere is organized for control of fine rapid movement like that which takes place in speaking. The non dominant hemisphere may well participate in generalized simple comprehension tasks but investigation of split brain patients (Gazzaniga and Sperry, 1965; Zaidel, 1978a, b) has shown that the left* hemisphere is superior in the perception and production of phonological elements. These studies have however all been concerned with segmental aspects of speech. The terms segmental and non segmental, express different but related aspects of speech production. *Segmental* is the basis for classification of actual sounds produced whereas *non segmental* refers to prosody, i.e. intonation, stress, pause, etc.

About non segmental features there is some ambivalence stemming in part from as yet insufficient knowledge. Prosody was at one time considered to be a right hemisphere function and indeed one regime of aphasia therapy is based on the possibility that framing speech in a melodic contour in some way activates the language areas in the non dominant hemisphere (Melodic Intonation Therapy, Sparks and Holland, 1976). An opposing view is that while certain non linguistic aspects of pitch, rhythm and loudness may be controlled by the right hemisphere, prosodic features are so intrinsic a part of the linguistic system that their properties belong to the left hemisphere (Robinson, 1977). The present writer has experience of a nine year-old boy who sustained right temperoparietal damage following a road accident. Conversational speech though somewhat slow in rate was generally appropriate prosodically. When asked to sing however, he intoned the tune with little variation in pitch or rhythm, though he was able to recognize well known tunes. Crystal (1981) in a footnote on the relationship between prosody and dominance makes the point that there is a difference between phonetic and phonological aspects and between affective and linguistic function. Affective states may be represented in the right hemisphere and also in subcortical structures particularly in the thalamus. Cerebellar dysfunction will produce phonetically based dysprosody in contrast to that which has a phonological basis and which is a feature of certain types of dysphasia and possibly of dyspraxia. In summary therefore, it is possible that prosody is a function of both cerebral hemispheres, and also of subcortical structures and the cerebellum but that the left hemisphere is dominant for linguistic function.

Localization

The standpoint of strict localization of function has given way latterly to a less rigid view of brain physiology. However, from evidence of cortical stimulation,

---

* For convenience the left hemisphere will be assigned dominance throughout the chapter.

from pathology and more recently from brain scan and blood flow studies, certain parts can be assigned specific functions with some degree of confidence. In relation to speech, the areas anterior and posterior to the Rolandic fissure are particularly concerned with movements necessary for articulation. The vocal tract is represented in the inferior part of the motor strip immediately above the Sylvian fissure. Organization and programming of speech is a function of Broca's area in the third frontal convolution and also of parts of the parietal area. Early literature while noting the anatomical siting of a supplementary motor area on the medial surface of the cerebral hemispheres ascribed little importance to it in relation to speech. More recent work, however, particularly that of Lassen and his colleagues (1978) indicates that this region is probably involved in ordering and sequential aspects of speech production (Fig. 1).

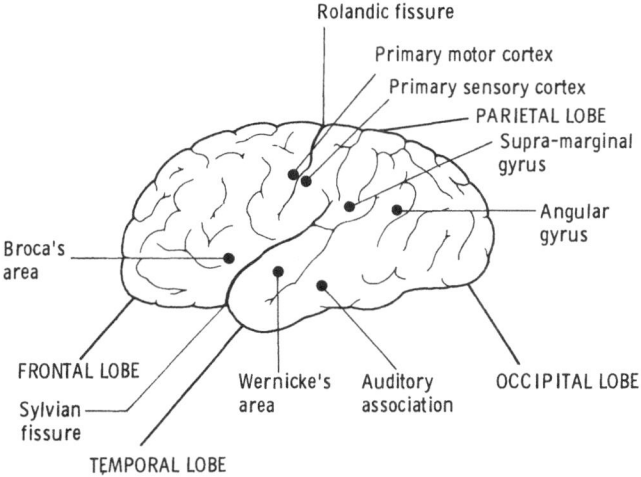

Fig. 1. Topography of cerebral hemispheres

Subcortically, the basal ganglia and the thalamic nuclei, particularly the ventrolateral nucleus of the thalamus are important relay stations in the integration, transmission and modification of information about speech production to and from the cerebral cortex.

The cerebellum exercises considerably monitoring control as do the nuclear masses in the mid brain and brain stem.

While therefore it is acceptable to assign specific functions to certain locations of the brain, it is also important in relation to speech production to regard each location as part of an integral whole which must function harmoniously. Lesions of one part of the central nervous system are likely to produce a ripple effect of dysfunction in other associated parts. In the ensuing more detailed description of the central and peripheral nervous systems, while there may be a focus on description of individual topography this overall concordance of function is implicit throughout the discussion.

Descending Supraspinal Systems

The main systems concerned with motor activity throughout the body have by tradition been known as the pyramidal and the extrapyramidal systems. However, Brodal (1981) calls into question many of the classically accepted views which have led to this labelling of motor systems.

In the first place, the concept of a purely motor function, he regards as erroneous since for many years it has been hypothesized, and more recent neurophysiological studies have established, that additional to their motor function, descending tracts exercise some control over ascending sensory impulses travelling to the brain. They also participate in reflexogenic activity within both the central and peripheral nervous system. From a clinical standpoint it is axiomatic that a separation of motor and sensory components of linguistic behaviour is in any case virtually impossible.

The term *pyramidal tract* Brodal (op.cit.) regards as in a strict sense only applying to that part of the descending pathway whose fibres form the pyramids, the *corticospinal tract*. Such a definition would exclude the descending fibres which pass to cranial nerve nuclei, *the corticobulbar tract*. However, because of recognized similarities between the two tracts, they are commonly designated as the pyramidal system, though it is important to recognize their separate identities.

There is however little ground for a similar treatment of the term *extrapyramidal system* and it is Brodal's view that: "neither theoretically nor practically is a useful purpose served by retaining the term *extrapyramidal*" (Brodal, 1981, p. 183).

Objection to the term stems from two sources: Firstly, it is unwieldy and gives rise to difficulties of delineation since theoretically it can encompass very many structures, lesions of which produce somewhat similar signs. Secondly, the term implies an entity which is discrete from the pyramidal system. The difficulty of separating the functions of descending systems is well recognized clinically and in the main, springs from their reciprocity through many inter-connections. Lesion studies have made apparent the near impossibility of assigning symptoms to any one specific site. In view of all this uncertainty about what is exactly entailed in this terminology it therefore would appear more apposite to use a general term such as *descending systems* and to identify each major one separately.

The Pyramidal System

Historically it was accepted that the origins of this pathway lay principally in the Betz cells of the prefrontal gyrus. Subsequent research has, however, revealed a discrepancy in that the number of fibres in the tract (in excess of 1,000,000) far exceeds the number of Betz cells in this region (between 25,000 and 30,000). It is thus apparent that only a small proportion of the fibres originate in this region. While an exact mapping of the origin of pyramidal fibres remains a task as yet not undertaken, various studies indicate some degree of consensus. The motor area (Brodman 4) provides the source of about 40% of the fibres. Here there is a somatotopical representation in which neurones subserving finely adjusted rapid movements such as take place in speech have a proportionately greater assigned area. About 20% of the fibres

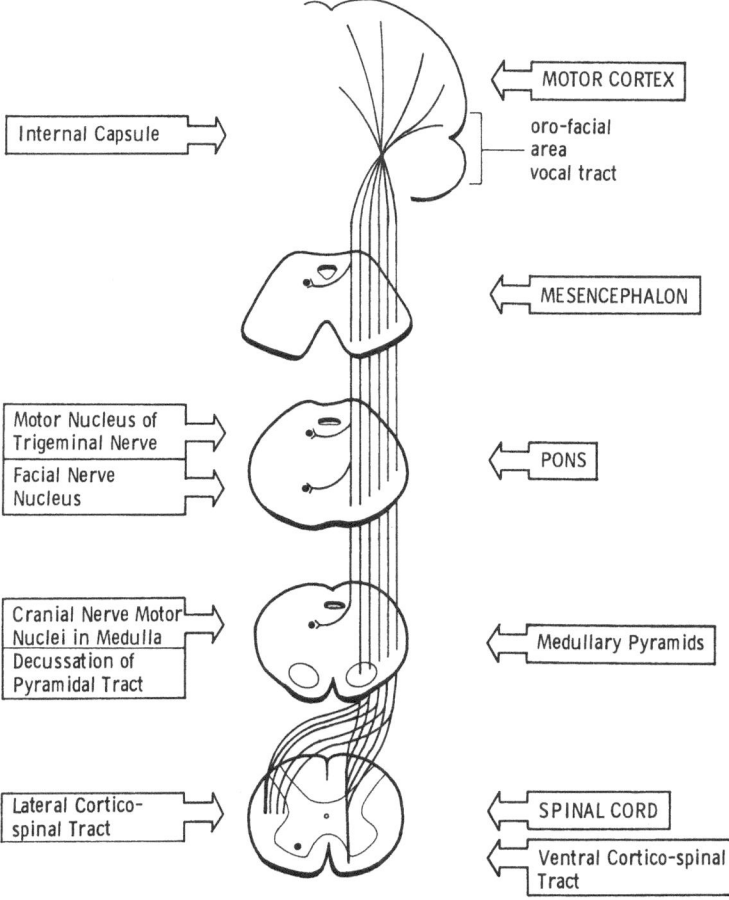

Fig. 2. Descending pathways in central nervous system, corticospinal and corticobulbar tracts

originate in the parietal lobe constituting the somesthetic cortex, thus giving further support to the concept of overlapping motor and sensory function. In fact, the particular area surrounding the central fissure is more accurately designated a *sensory motor area* since its function appears to be one of integration.

The remaining fibres originate in the premotor cortex anterior to the motor area, the posterior part of the parietal lobe and in the supplementary motor area which lies on the medial surface of the hemisphere adjacent and anterior to the paracentral lobule.

The fibres of the pyramidal system show considerable variation in diameter and consequently in the velocity with which impulses are conducted. The largest myelinated fibres are probably the axons of the giant Betz cells and these have the highest velocity. About 60% of all the fibres are myelinated, the remaining 40% being slow acting fibres whose function is thought to be concerned with central transmission of sensory impulses and with some spinal reflexes (Brodal, op.cit.).

Corticospinal Tract

From the cortex, the tract transverses the *corona radiata* and passes through the posterior limb of the *internal capsule*. Here it is in intimate association with other tracts travelling to subcortical relay stations. There is evidence, however, that the fibres to some extent retain a somatotopic distribution determined by their cells of origin. In the peduncles of the midbrain there is separation because of intercalation of the nuclear masses but beyond this they unite again to form the pyramids of the *medulla oblongata*. At this point the majority, about 85%, of the fibres cross over and continue as the *lateral corticospinal tract* in the dorsal lateral white column of the spinal cord. Here in the grey matter they nearly all terminate on internuncial neurones which in turn synapse with alpha and gamma neurones. Distribution of terminating fibres reflects a proportionately higher ratio of innervation in the cervical area; 55%, with the thoracic area receiving 20% of fibres and the lumbosacral area 25%.

A small number of pyramidal fibres which do not cross continue as the *ventral corticospinal tract*. This terminates in the anterior horn of the spinal cord in the cervical and upper thoracic regions. Together with a few uncrossed fibres which travel in the lateral corticospinal tract (ipsilateral) it contributes to the bilateral innervation of cervical and thoracic musculature (see Fig. 2).

Along its path, the corticospinal tract gives off a number of collateral branches. The principal ones are:

from the axons of the Betz cells back to the cortex where their function is assumed to be connected with activation and inhibition of adjacent areas,

to the striate body,
to the substantia nigra,
to the red nucleus,
to the reticular formation, and
to the pontile nuclei (Guyton, 1972).

It should, however, be noted that recent studies cited by Brodal (op.cit.), in which the enzyme Horseradish peroxidase (HRP) has been used to trace pathways, indicate additionally, independent connections directly between the cortex and the subcortical relay stations. This fact suggests that the latter are less reliant on the corticospinal tract than has been traditionally assumed.

Corticobulbar Tract

This pursues a similar course to the corticospinal tract through the internal capsule and peduncles. Thereafter bundles of fibres branch off periodically to synapse within the motor nuclei of the cranial nerves in the brain stem. These will be considered in further detail in the section on the peripheral nervous system, below. Many of the fibres of the corticobulbar tract cross over in the brain stem so that control of cranial nerve musculature is in part contralateral. There is, however, some ipsilateral innervation so that a unilateral lesion will not necessarily lead to a complete paralysis though there may well be a weakness of movement.

Functions of the Pyramidal System

Because of its intimate association with a number of other pathways, delineation of precise function is difficult. On these grounds Brodal (op. cit.) advocates discontinuation of the term *pyramidal tract syndrome*. There is certainly no defined link between individual cortical cells and specific movements. Possible models of motor function will be discussed in more detail in Chapter 4.

It is now thought that the chief contribution of the pyramidal system lies in the development of the skill and agility necessary to carry out discrete voluntary movement. Denny Brown (1966) thought that the pyramidal system was much concerned with necessary adjustments which could adapt movement accurately to the demands of the stimulus. Lesions may produce impairment of this ability so that, for example, in relation to speech there is a failure to differentiate between degrees of force of movement appropriate to differing types of articulation. In some types of "upper motor neurone" dysarthria, speech may be described as explosive and is indicative of over prolonged contact between articulators.

Other Descending Pathways

The chief of these are the rubrospinal, the reticulospinal, the vestibulospinal and the tectospinal tracts. They serve to connect lower motor neurones with subcortical and indirectly with cortical structures. Both the reticular formation and the red nucleus have direct connections with the cerebral cortex through the corticoreticular and the corticorubral tracts. They also receive fibres from the cerebellum and from the substantia nigra.

These pathways descending to the spinal cord and to nuclei of cranial nerves constitute important links in the transmission of information from cortical and subcortical structures.

The vestibular nuclei through the vestibular spinal tract connect with the grey matter in the anterior horn of the spinal cord. Through ascending pathways there is distribution to the nuclei of the abducens, trochlear and oculomotor cranial nerves. Mediated through the vestibular nerve, the vestibulospinal tract serves to maintain balance and to coordinate head and eye movement. The tectospinal tract is also concerned with the coordination of eye movement.

Striate Body (Basal Ganglia)

These is a group of nuclei which exercise an important role in the control of motor speech. As well as constituting a system of relay stations whereby, indirectly, the cerebral cortex is enabled to exert influence on motor activity, they are now recognized as having a much wider range of function.

There is some divergence of view as to what properly constitutes the "basal ganglia" and in the past the thalamus, for example, has been included under this heading. Clinically the substantia nigra is often included with the striate body as part of the basal ganglia. In the present context the term *striate body* (basal ganglia) serves as a collective name for the following paired nuclei (Fig. 3):

    caudate nucleus,
    putamen,
    globus pallidus, and
    claustrum.

The putamen and globus pallidus are also referred to as the *lenticular nucleus.* Closely associated with the striate body are:

    the amygdaloid nucleus,
    the thalamus,
    the subthalamic nuclei,
    the substantia nigra, and
    the red nucleus.

The basal ganglia appear to be part of an interconnecting circuit between the cerebral cortex and the thalamus. Barr (1979) suggests that this circuit has an important regulatory influence on movement and that it is especially well developed in man. Present evidence indicates a poorly developed connection between the basal ganglia and brain stem structures. Other connections are with the substantia nigra and the subthalamic nuclei. The caudate and lenticular (putamen and globus pallidus) nuclei are composed of interconnecting neurones. They receive cortico fugal fibres originating in all major parts of the cerebral cortex. They also receive afferent fibres from the thalamic nuclei and from the substantia nigra. The globus pallidus is the main efferent nucleus. Its principal connection is to the thalamus which in turn connects with the motor area of the cortex thus completing the loop connection mentioned above.

The *substantia nigra* which is very well developed in man has a distinctive appearance characterized by its dark colour. This is due to the interspersion of the pigment melanin. The nigrostriatal pathway is of considerable importance because of its dopaminergic function. Dopamine acts as a neurotransmitter and it is thought that the onset of certain dyskinetic conditions like Parkinson's disease arises from the destruction of the dopamine producing cells, in the substantia nigra. A review by Iverson (1975), however, indicates that dopamine has connections with a number of disorders other than Parkinson's

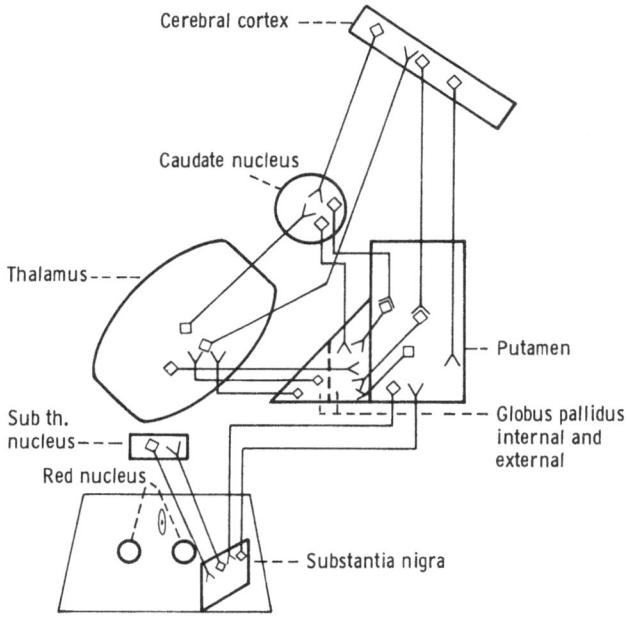

Fig. 3. Schematic representation of basal ganglia and their connections

disease; schizophrenia is one example (see Chapter 5). It seems also that while the nigrostriatal projection is the most readily recognized, in fact it may well be only one of several in the dopaminergic system. There are other neurotransmitters in the substantia nigra; a substance "P" and another, GABA have been cited. Their function in the brain is not known at present but they may well be responsible for some aspects of kinesis. The substantia nigra has a direct link with the thalamus, thus again demonstrating indirect influence upon the motor area of the cerebral cortex.

Thalamus

Reference has been made to the ascending connections between the thalamus and cerebral cortex; there are also descending pathways. The close association between these two regions of the brain has led to the suggestion that the cortex may almost be regarded as an outgrowth of the thalamus (Guyton, 1972). A mapping of cortical and thalamic areas appears to suggest common functions. In relation to speech, the thalamus is traditonally regarded as part of the central language system and thus, thalamic dysfunction has been associated with dysphasic type disorders. But it also appears to exercise some control over motor speech. The lateral ventral nucleus in particular may influence non segmental aspects of speech relating to timing and ordering as well as to resonatory and phonatory parameters. Bell (1968) reported on patients who had undergone thalamotomies. In 38 out of 59 cases there were postoperative changes in speech production. A number of these suffered dysarthric type disorders which persisted after concomitant limb pareses had remitted. Geschwind (1967) also described a similar type of disorder as a sequel of thalamic surgery. Myers (1967) referred to evoked response studies which demonstrated reciprocal discharges in pyramidal tract neurones following stimulation of the ventrolateral thalamic nucleus. Indirectly, of course, the thalamus has a significant and wide reaching effect upon speech since all sensory pathways (excluding olfactory) pass through it to the cortex. Through the reticular system it is also implicated in mechanisms of attention which facilitate specific types of mental activity.

The Reticular System. Red Nucleus

Throughout the medulla oblongata and pons there is a network of ascending and descending fibres, in which are embedded many cell masses. These are the reticular nuclei. They receive and project fibres which connect with the spinal cord, the motor nuclei of cranial nerves, the cerebellum and the basal ganglia.

The red nucleus which lies in the midbrain through the corticorubral tract receives fibres from the motor and premotor regions of the cerebral cortex as does the reticular formation via the corticoreticular tract. Both form part of a feedback circuit through their respective relationship with the cerebellum.

The reticular formation exercises control over discrete movement through the gamma reflex loop. It is likely that its function is concerned with maintenance of appropriate levels of muscular tension throughout the body including the vocal tract (Rhines and Magoun, 1946). Through its ascending pathways it provides sensory information to the cerebellum and is thus indirectly concerned with mediation of motor activity.

Cerebellar System

The function of the cerebellum appears to be one of programming and control of movement rather than that of initiation. This role has far reaching implications in relation to disorders of speech production where an impairment in the motor programming function is central to the understanding of their nature. Brodal (op.cit.) suggests that because of the multiplicity of its connections the cerebellum is able to exert influence on almost any part of the brain.

The cerebellum acts as a tuner and a modifier of motor schemata. It is known that the cerebral cortex issues motor commands in excess of those required for the accomplishment of specific movements; this excess may well be modified in the cerebellum.

There is a wide disparity in the ratio of input to output fibres, something of the order of 40 : 1. Numerically the proportion of efferent fibres is about 5% of that of afferents. This gives some indication of the importance of its role in terms of refinement and modification of motor programmes.

The cerebellum is divided into two major lobes which are connected through a central part, the vermis.

Anatomically the cerebellum consists of a surface layer of deeply convoluted grey matter. These convolutions form transverse bands across its surface (folia). Its central part is composed of white matter representing intracerebellar connections as well as those which connect with other parts of the brain. Buried deep in the white matter are four pairs of nuclei: fastigeal, globose, emboliform and a large irregular shaped nucleus which is most prominently developed in man; this is the dentate nucleus.

The cerebellar cortex histologically is made up of complex but very precisely patterned cellular arrays. Essentially it may be divided into three layers, the molecular, that which contains the large Purkinje cells and the granular layer. The molecular layer which has relatively few nerve cells consists mainly of nerve fibres representing dendritic branches of the Purkinje cells and axons from cells in the granular layer. These cells are stellate in form; one particular type is the basket cell, so called because of the form in which collaterals from their axons configurate around the dendrites of the Purkinje cells to synapse with them.

The Purkinje layer takes its name from the large flask shaped cells which are arranged throughout in a regular manner. These give off complex branched dendrites into the molecular layer. Their axons project to the cerebellar nuclei. To ensure maximum synaptic contact, the dendrites are profusely covered with spines estimated to be about 100,000 on each one. The axons of the Purkinje cells project into the central white matter. Axons of Purkinje cells provide the only efferent projection in the cerebellum. Their function is inhibitory.

The granular layer is composed of densely packed small neurones. Their axons ascend to the molecular layer where they branch in a T formation, running longitudinally and parallel to the folia. A second type of cell, a Golgi cell, also projects into the molecular layer. There are two types of afferents to the cerebellar cortex. These are climbing fibres and mossy fibres. Climbing fibres have a special relationship with Purkinje cells. The majority originate in the inferior olive though some are thought to come from other parts of the brain, possibly the pontine nuclei and the reticular formation. These fibres transverse the white matter of the cerebellum and synapse principally with the Purkinje cells by branching profusely in a vine-like manner.

Mossy fibres form the largest number of afferents. These thick myelinated fibres terminate by synapsing with the granular cells. Towards their terminal points the fibres develop numerous small swellings called rosettes. Configurations of these rosettes, synapses of granular cells and axons of Golgi cells together form a *glomerulus*.

Afferent Connections. The pontine nuclei are the most important relay stations between the cerebral cortex and the cerebellum. Phylogenetically they show increasingly complex structure and are at their most highly developed state in man. They receive fibres from the corticopontine tract which has its origins in all four main lobes of the cerebral hemispheres. The tract descends adjacent to the corticospinal tract to end in a circumscribed somatotopical arrangement in the ipsilateral pontine nucleus. It is probable that the corticospinal tract also gives off collaterals to the pontine nuclei, but a number of studies (e.g. Allen, Korn, Oshima and Toyama, 1975), lend support to the view that activation of cells in the pontine nuclei is probably mediated through the separate and direct fibres of the corticopontine tract. Axons of the pontine nuclei travel along the contralateral middle cerebellar peduncle (brachium pontis). They enter the cerebellum and are distributed throughout the cortex where they end as mossy fibres (Fig. 4a).

The inferior cerebellar peduncle (restiform and juxta restiform body) consists of fibres from the inferior olive, the spinocerebellar tracts, the reticular formation and the vestibular system. Afferents from the sensory trigeminal nucleus have also been described (Brodal, op.cit.). The fibres are distributed throughout the cortex, those originating in the inferior olive terminating as climbing fibres which synapse with the Purkinje cells.

Efferent Connections. The main output from the cerebellum is by way of the superior cerebellar peduncle. Axons of neurones leave the four main nuclei. Their chief target is the thalamus and in particular the ventrolateral nucleus. There they synapse with neurones which connect with the cerebral cortex, principally the motor area. Other efferent pathways leave the cerebellum for the reticular formation, the vestibular nuclei and the red nucleus (Figs. 4b and c).

Each of the paired cerebellar nuclei has circumscribed functions and some of these have been delineated in experimental animals. In man, however, where evidence is usually deduced from pathological conditions, the position is by no means so clear, since rarely does it happen that damage to one structure does not influence function in adjacent parts. It seems possible that the dentate nucleus with its direct connection to the thalamus may play a vital part in speech production. Larson, Sutton and Lindemann (1978) have demonstrated the effect of cerebellar lesions on respiratory and laryngeal neurology which indicates that the anterior lobes are implicated in laryngeal control.

The cerebellum is a key structure in a number of feedback systems. Afferent impulses from the cerebral cortex, from spinocerebellar tracts and from cranial nerves bring in information which is processed and modified in a manner still little understood before being returned to the cerebral cortex via the thalamic nuclei. This feedback loop is to some extent influenced by external events. Internal feedback circuits are provided through the pontine-cerebellar-pontine pathways, the reticular-cerebellar-reticular pathways and the cerebellar-thalamic-cortical-cerebellar route. The last named is an extremely rapid circuit. Bloomfield and Marr (1970) discussing cerebellar function quote a time of between 6 and 10 ms for completion of the whole circuit. Through this route the cerebellum is able to monitor and control all

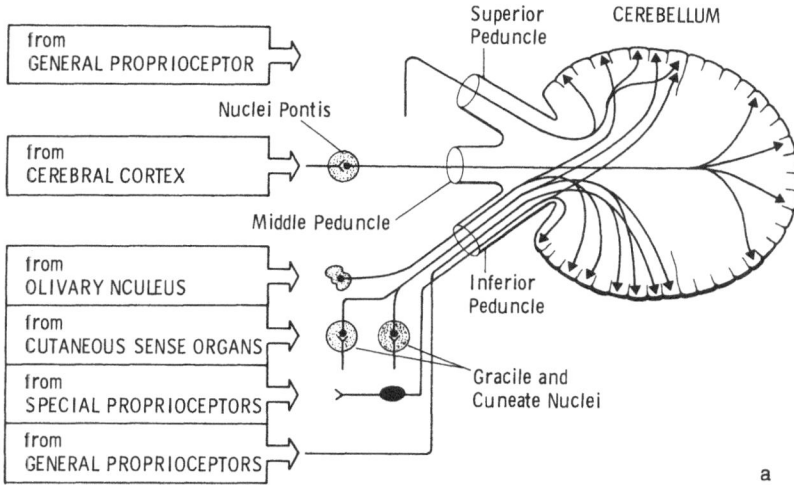

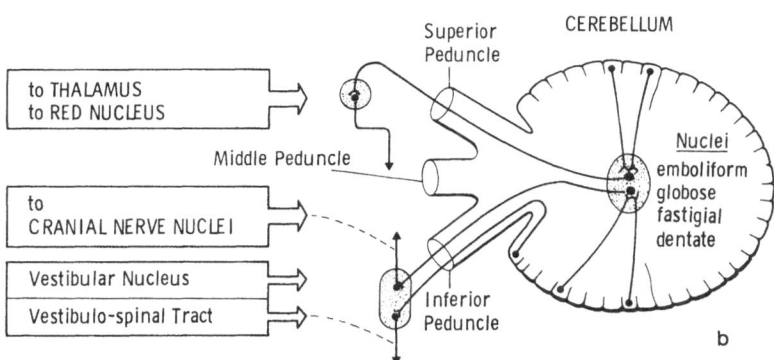

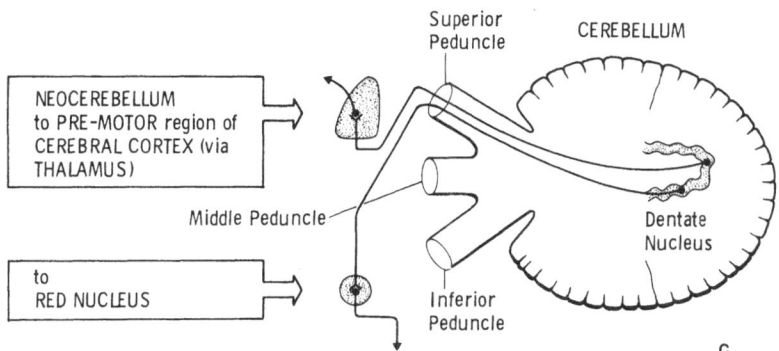

Fig. 4. *a* Afferent pathways to cerebellum, *b, c* efferent pathways from cerebellum. (After McNaught, A., Callender, R.: Illustrated Physiology. Edinburgh: E. & S. Livingstone)

pyramidal tract activity. It operates as an integrator of diverse movements creating a harmonious whole. In its monitoring role it compares incoming information with that which is already recognized and intended, and facilitates necessary corrections at the level of the cerebral cortex. Lesions of the cerebellar tissue result in devastating disintegration of movement and this includes articulatory gestures. There is a marked difficulty both in initiating and in terminating speech, and length, stress, and pitch are all grossly affected. The skill with which we are enabled to carry out integrated movements becomes for the most part automatic and it is only when dysfunction occurs that there is realization of the complexity involved. Eccles (1973) contends that the cerebellum is the seat of all this immensely complicated movement and "that throughout life and particularly in the early years we are engaged in an incessant teaching program for the cerebellum" (p. 123). Impairment of cerebellar function will affect rapid movement most markedly. In this respect it is complementary to the basal ganglia which are thought to be concerned more with coordination of slow movement.

Each cerebellar hemisphere influences movement on the ipsilateral side of the body because of decussation of fibres ascending to the cerebral cortex.

Kent and Netsell (1975) advance three possibilities regarding the role of the cerebellum in the execution of skilled movement. The first is the facilitation of information received from muscle spindles to higher centres as a movement is carried out. Interruption of this information will result in a lack of proprioceptive feedback so that necessary adjustments in velocity and muscle tone do not take place. The second possibility is that the cerebellum acting as a coordinator of incoming information exercises control over the timing and direction of movement. Third is the modification of cortical motor commands through the cerebro-cerebellar loop "the refining function" described by Eccles. Kornhuber (1974) also suggests that the cerebral cortex does not set up a precise temporal programme of the whole movement but provides only a general indication of sequence which is then executed in a step by step fashion under the timing control of the cerebellum. This view has considerable relevance when we come later to consider the theory of motor equivalence as it relates to articulatory programming.

Brodal (op.cit.) stresses the marked ability for compensation which characterizes cerebellar lesions. This is particularly evident in children and adolescents where some plasticity of brain function is still retained. Whether compensation is the result of other systems assuming the role of the cerebellum or whether intact parts take over function of damaged areas is not known.

The Peripheral Nervous System

This description focusses on the innervation of skeletal musculature directly involved in speech production and on the particular manner whereby control is exercised through feedback circuits. A comprehensive account of feedback processes would include detailed description of auditory and, though to a lesser extent, visual pathways. However, such consideration lies beyond the scope of the present work and will therefore only be included insofar as it relates to motor function. The term "peripheral" refers to all nervous pathways which lie outside the central nervous system and, in the case of cranial nerves, to their nuclei in the brain stem.

Transmission

Transmission of impulses along nervous pathways is an electrochemical process which entails shifts between negative and positive charges within nerve fibres. Such shifts are brought about by a complex interchange of ions through the axonal membrane. Specifically, potassium and sodium ions interchange following excitation of the nerve fibre thus facilitating the flow of current in a series of impulses. These are action potentials. Where the flow is along unmyelinated fibres it is smooth and continuous but where they are myelinated flow is saltatory, that is to say, it proceeds in a series of "jumps". Myelination provides for good insulation and this would normally inhibit the flow of current brought about by the ionisation process but this is circumvented by an interruption of the myelin sheath at regular intervals along the fibre. These junctures are called the *Nodes of Ranvier* and it is at these points that the interchange of ions takes place. Myelination allows for a much more rapid conductance of impulses. There is a considerable variation in the velocity of conduction throughout the nervous system. In the case of small unmyelinated fibres it may be as low as 0.5 m per second, while large myelinated fibres may be able to transmit at speeds of up to 130 m per second (Guyton, 1972). Most of the cranial nerves which subserve the musculature of the vocal tract are myelinated so that rapid transport of commands from the central nervous system for execution of precise movements can be effected. The strength of muscle contraction depends on the frequency *of firing* of impulses and it is also influenced by the actual number of motor units activated.

The Motor Neurone

Control over striated muscle is brought about through the action of motor neurones. Within each bundle of fibres are parallel fibres which are collected together in spindle shaped structures to form special receptor endings: *the muscle spindles.* The fibres forming the spindles are called intrafusal to differentiate them from the extrafusal fibres of the main muscle (Figs. 5a and b).

Each motor neurone supplies a number of muscle fibres and the neurone and the fibres it supplies are collectively called *the motor unit.* For musculature where fine delicate action is required, the innervation ratio is high, each motor neurone supplying only a few fibres; for gross movement it is much lower. Contraction of muscle is brought about through a further electrochemical

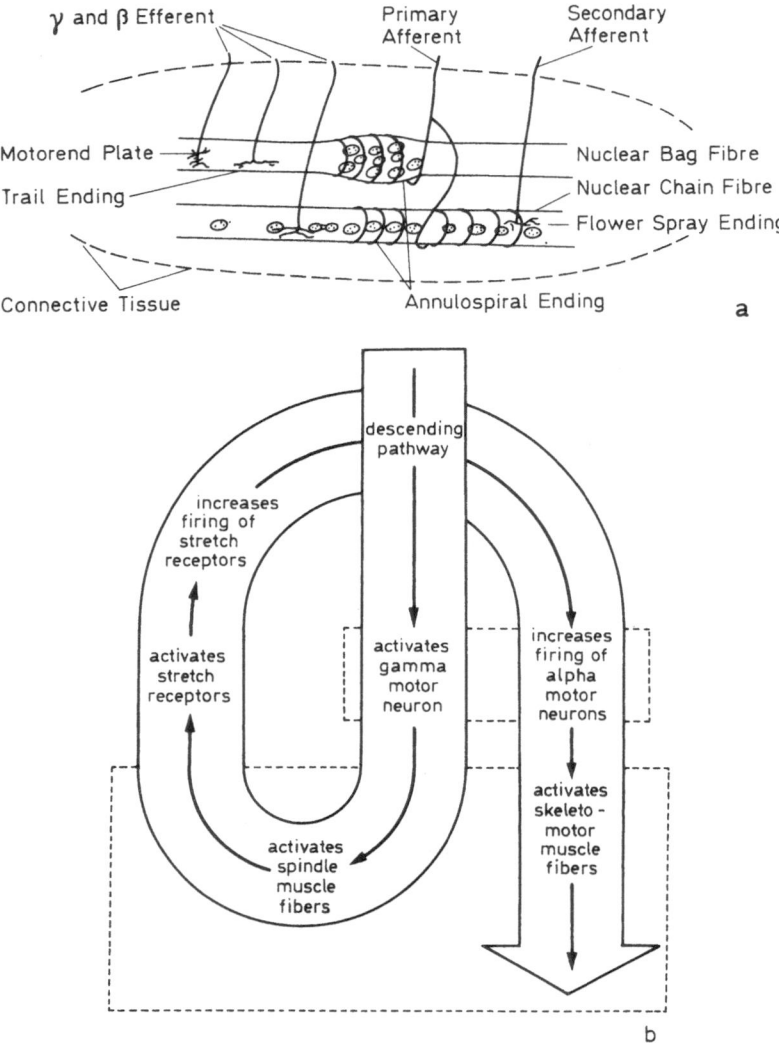

Fig. 5. *a* Diagram of muscle spindle, *b* Gamma loop. The small rectangle at the center indicates those effects occurring in the brainstem or spinal cord; the large rectangle, the effects in the muscle. (Fig. 5 b reproduced from: Luciano, D., Vandver, A. J., Sherman, J. H.: Human Structure and Function. McGraw-Hill. 1978)

process which takes place at the juncture of terminal branches of the nerve fibre and the muscle fibres, *the motor end plate*. Acetylcholine is released and diffused across the membrane of the motor end plate facilitating the passage of ions. The potential of the muscle fibres is changed and when this reaches a critical state of depolarization inception of muscular contraction comes about. Initially each fibre contracts once, but for effective contraction to take place there must be repetitive stimulation of fibres so that the summation of individual motor unit activity produces a smooth sustained contraction (tetanic contraction). To produce appropriate gradation of movement it is obvious that the motor units must not work on an all-or-none basis. They have differing thresholds of excitation so that firing is not necessarily in synchrony. Together with tetanization this ensures smooth muscular contraction regardless of its degree of force.

Control over muscle contraction is brought about by reflex action involving the muscle spindles. Each spindle is enclosed in a sheath of connective tissue and contains between two and ten individual fibres. These are of two types. In one, the middle part, is expanded and its nuclei are clustered together in this region. This is the *nuclear bag*. The other type, called the *nuclear chain,* as the name implies, has its nuclei strung out along the length of the fibre. A further division of the nuclear bag type, bag_1 and bag_2, has recently been proposed. The differentiation is based on chemical and structural factors and also on different function.

Muscle spindles are innervated by afferent and efferent fibres. The afferent supply is from large A-group fibres whose terminal portion winds round the central body of the intrafusal fibre in a spiral manner; this ending is known as an *annulospiral* or primary ending. There are also secondary endings. These are smaller in diameter and end in arborizing filaments known as *flower spray endings.* Annulo spiral endings are usually found on both nuclear bag and chain fibres whereas flower spray endings tend to be seen only on nuclear chain fibres.

The efferent nerve supply (an unusual feature in a sensory end organ) is by gamma fibres (fusimotor) which are distributed as motor end plates and also as diffuse trail endings at the distal parts of the fibre (Brodal, 1981).

The central parts of the intrafusal fibres are incapable of contraction but stimulation by the gamma supply will cause the ends to contract with subsequent stretching of the medial part and consequent stimulation of the sensory endings.

For many years it was thought that muscle spindles were mainly concerned only with the monitoring of length, in contrast to tendon organs whose chief function was to record contraction. It is now thought that they have an additional function related to the recording of velocity of stretch. Information about length provides the *static response* and recent work (e.g. Boyd, 1976) indicates that bag_2 and chain fibres are responsible for this while *dynamic response* concerned with velocity originates in bag_1 fibres. Secondary endings appear to share similar functions with primary endings but are slower to respond. The two types of gamma endings mentioned above appear to mediate the two types of response, end plates the dynamic, and trail endings the static type. The contribution of muscle spindles to movement is reflexogenic. Stretching of the muscle activates the sensory endings within the spindles causing them to fire impulses along the 1a afferent fibres. The afferents synapse with alpha motor neurones in the spinal cord or in the cranial nerve nuclei, which in turn cause the extrafusal fibres to contract. The spindle afferents then become desensitized. This stretch reflex is absolutely essential for the maintenance of muscle tone throughout the body. It ensures the body being able to preserve a state of equilibrium in varying conditions.

There are many different types of reflex activity and this stretch reflex represents one of the most simple. Its elicitation as in the knee jerk forms a routine part of clinical neurological investigation.

The gamma loop is also subject to influence from higher cortical centres. Impulses travelling down the corticospinal and corticobulbar tracts synapse with the gamma motor neurones reinforcing the activation of the sensory endings in the muscle spindles (Fig. 5b).

Muscle spindles also indirectly play a part in coordination of movement through afferent connections with the cerebellum and to a lesser extent with the sensori motor cortex.

Tendon organs have an opposing function to muscle spindles. Their structure is much less complex and essentially they consist of groups of myelinated nerve fibres whose fine endings are interspersed among tendinous tissue. They detect activity within muscle fibres associated with increased tension. Through afferent connections they are able to exercise an inhibitory action on alpha motor neurones thus producing relaxation of the muscle. They act in reciprocal relationship to muscle spindles. This guards against damage to muscles.

These two sensory endings constitute important elements in control of movement. Less well studied has been the influence of *joint receptors*. In the context of speech production the role of these receptors particularly with reference to those found in the tempero mandibular joint and in the larynx is likely to be of paramount importance. They have been described by Wyke and his colleagues (e.g. Wyke, 1967; Klineberg, Greenfield and Wyke, 1970). Four different morphological types of ending have been delineated within joint capsules. These are types 1–4. The first three are encapsulated endings, while type 4, comprising small unmyelinated fibres is free ending. These mechanoreceptors exert a powerful influence on musculature. Wyke (1967) and Freeman and Wyke (1967) interpret types 1 and 2 as being concerned with jaw position and speed of movement while types 3 and 4 are more likely to be activated by pathological conditions and may therefore function as pain receptors.

The close relationship of jaw movement to speech is obvious and it has been assumed that the visceral activity of mastication has a direct connection with the development of speech articulation. The establishment of "good" feeding patterns forms a cornerstone of some types of speech therapy with cerebral palsied children. However, an opposing view is discussed in Chapter 4.

In the light of recent work to be discussed further in Chapter 3, there may well be a case for a specificity of motor programming as it relates to speech. Earlier work (Miller and Hardy, 1962) indicates a need to consider a differential approach to speech related and non speech movement of oral structures. This of course applies to upper motor neurone pathology where it is the programming element which is impaired (see Chapter 4).

Joint receptors have somewhat confusingly been labelled as Ruffini endings and Pacinian corpuscles because they bear a resemblance to those endings found in other parts of the body. This nomenclature is not advocated.

Meissner's corpuscles are another type of ending also concerned with speech. They are found in the perioral region and in the tongue. They are extremely sensitive to minute changes in pressure and as such may well play an important part in fine adjustments to ensure precision of articulation.

Touch and pressure is also mediated through *end bulbs* distributed throughout the subcutaneous region of the mouth.

Hardcastle (1976) draws attention to the possible significance of periodontal receptors. These are free ending filaments distributed throughout the periodontal membrane. He suggests that their high degree of sensitivity may play a part in the fine control of articulation.

Muscle spindles and tendon organs are found throughout all the tissues connected with speech production.

The distribution of end organs within the oral region is not even. In some parts they are clustered together while in others they are more sparsely distributed. End organs concerned with recognition of positioning (proprioceptors) are, for example, more densely aggregated in the anterior parts of the tongue, with a more scattered occurrence towards the dorsal part (Dixon, 1962).

Feedback

The role of feedback as a part of the neurolinguistic programming of speech will be discussed more fully in the next chapter. Neurophysiologically, however, it is apparent that there must be an efficient link between the receiver and the transmitter both for the integration of incoming information and for monitoring of action.

Peripherally, feedback is effected through auditory, visual and tactile channels. These are exteroceptive. Interoceptive feedback arises from within the body and is usually known as *proprioception*. These channels provide information during ongoing speech about muscle tension and position and about speech and direction of movement. Hardcastle (op.cit.) lists the differing types and properties of feedback circuits involved in speech production. Tactile feedback which gives information about time duration and location of pressure and contact is a slowly acting circuit. Information from this source reaches the central nervous system *after* the event. Proprioceptors on the other hand provide rapid transmission of feedback. They transmit information about length and rate of stretch, direction and extent of movement. This is conveyed both *before* and *during* the movement so that a predictive function can be incorporated in any preprogramming activity relating to speech. Auditory feedback provides information *after* the event. By its very nature of conduction through sound waves it is the slowest acting of all the channels.

Speech is also monitored visually and of course this and tactile proprioception are the main channels enabling deafened people to maintain and understand speech. The role of auditory perception and visual perception lies outside the scope of this particular book and will not be discussed in detail.

Proprioceptive and tactile feedback take place throughout the vocal tract and as such exercise a wide influence. It is difficult to consider any one parameter of speech production without reference to its close relationship with others. Respiratory action, phonation, resonance and articulation influence each other continuously in ongoing speech.

Much of this feedback is at unconscious level and is not under direct voluntary control. Wyke (e.g. 1970, 1974) has made extensive contributions to our views of reflexive feedback in laryngeal musculature. He has demonstrated the ways in which feedback from mechanoreceptor systems interact with egressive air streams to control vocal fold movement. Downstream in the articulatory mechanisms it is also likely that some ongoing adjustments are at an unconscious level too, since the speed with which alteration and modification of movement is carried out precludes any conscious intervention from the central nervous system particularly once the sequence of movements is learned.

Thus speech is facilitated and controlled at different levels by extremely complex servo systems: at an unconscious level through muscle spindle and tendon reflex loops and at central level through intervention by the cerebellum, basal ganglia and within the various neuronal pools which have been described. Structures within the central nervous system exercise influence on peripheral parts mainly through the gamma efferent loop.

Evidence about the effect of interruption of proprioceptive and tactile pathways on speech is conflicting, partly because this is a difficult function to investigate in man. Stereognostic tasks are inconclusive and it has been shown that many adequate speakers have poor oral stereognostic function, while adequate discrimination has been demonstrated in speakers with marked disorders (Macdonald and Aungst, 1970). Blocking of the mandibular branch of the trigeminal nerve has been attempted to assess the effect of inhibition of proprioceptive feedback. This of course also affects efferent pathways, but Abbs (1973) suggested that as these were composed of larger fibres they would recover before the smaller gamma sensory fibres thus producing a selective cut off of proprioceptors. Results showed that jaw movement was noticeably slower but there was not a marked effect on speech. Other studies involving sensory deprivation (e.g. Gammon, Smith, Daniloff and Kim, 1971) have demonstrated changes in articulatory patterns particularly in the ability to make fine gradations in movement as for example in production of complex sounds like affricates [tʃ] and [dʒ].

Cranial Nerves

To understand something of the way in which the central nervous system exercises control over the vocal tract and also to attempt an understanding of the ways whereby information is carried from the periphery, integrated and acted upon, some discussion of the part played by relevant cranial nerves is necessary (Fig. 6).

Motor control of speech musculature is under the influence of the following cranial nerves:

Trigeminal CN V, Facial CN VII, Glossopharyngeal CN IX, Vagus CN X, Hypoglossal CN XII.

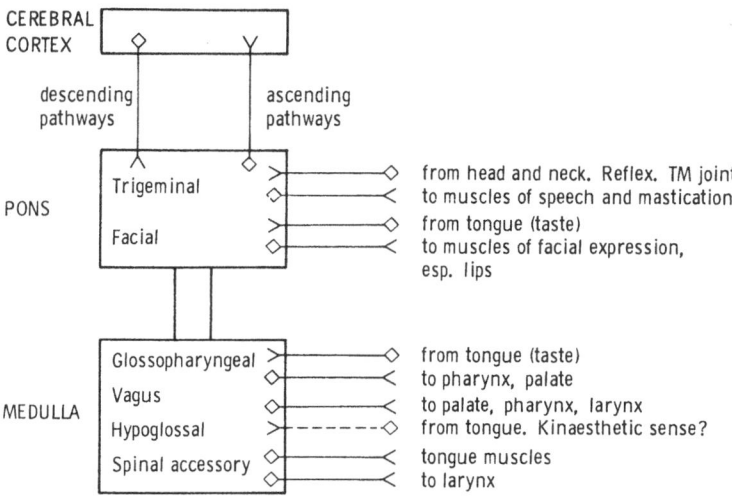

Fig. 6. Schematic representation of peripheral nervous system

Of course, other cranial nerves play some part and notably the VIIIth (acoustic and vestibular) is essential for speech as indeed are those controlling respiratory activity, but a discussion of their role is not included here.

Cranial nerve nuclei both sensory and motor have complex interconnecting relations with many parts of the central nervous system other than their main destinations in the sensory cortex and the periphery respectively. The *trigeminal nerve* is mixed having both motor and sensory fibres. Its motor components innervate inter alia, facial muscles involved in mastication and in speech. It also projects fibres to the tensor palati and tensor tympani as well as to the anterior part of the digastric muscles. The motor nucleus lies adjacent to the main sensory trigeminal nucleus in the pons. This is acted upon by descending fibres (crossed) of the corticobulbar tract, by reflexive connections with sensory trigeminal nuclei and also by afferents from other cranial nerves.

The sensory component of the trigeminal nerve is considerably larger than its motor branch. Its function is mainly concerned with transmission of general sensation from cutaneous parts of the head, face, nasal and oral mucosa. The afferent trigeminal complex is also responsible for the myotatic reflex and for the articular reflex systems which maintain temperomandibular posture (Wyke, 1974).

Trigeminal nuclei are three intercommunicating structures, *the chief sensory nucleus,* caudally the *nucleus of the trigeminal spinal tract* and the *mesencephalic nucleus.* The chief sensory nucleus is thought to send nearly all its ascending fibres to the thalamus (Brodal, op. cit.) and presumably thence indirectly through further connections to the sensory cortex via the thalamocortical tracts. It is particularly concerned with discrimination of touch.

A number of sensory root fibres course along the spinal trigeminal tract together with fibres from the facial, glossopharyngeal and vagus nerves. They terminate in the spinal nucleus a long structure lying adjacent to the tract. As the tract descends, branches are given off to different parts of the nucleus. At its caudal end it is indistinguishable from the grey matter of the dorsal horn of the spinal cord in its cervical region. The spinal nucleus is thought to receive afferents yielding information about pain and temperature, but apart from these somewhat general functions very little is understood.

The third trigeminal nucleus, the mesencephalic, is probably concerned with the mediation of kinaesthetic input arising in joint receptors, muscle spindles and tendon organs. Its axons are in close association with the mandibular nerve. Others are connected with the alveolar nerves and appear sensitive to pressure in the periodontal area.

The trigeminal nuclei, as well as sending fibres to the reticular formation also project to the cerebellum via the inferior cerebellar peduncle. Lesions of peripheral parts of the trigeminal nerve may result in a reduction or loss of sensation in the facial area. Damage to the motor component will produce a unilateral or bilateral paresis or paralysis of masticatory muscles. Mandibular movement will be impaired and the patient may be required to adopt compensatory oral gestures in order to chew, bite and to speak intelligibly.

Another very distressing and painful condition associated with this nerve is that of trigeminal neuralgia. Its aetiology is not well understood at present.

The facial nerve is also a mixed nerve, its motor roots being the most important. These are responsible for innervation of the muscles of facial expression (e.g. obicularis, oris, buccinator) and also the stapedius muscle, the stylohyoid and the posterior belly of the digastric muscle.

Brodal (op. cit.) states that very little is known about the afferent innervation of muscles of facial expression. It would be reasonable to assume that they are endowed with proprioceptors but very few muscle spindles have been found in human tissue.

The motor nucleus is influenced by several sources and in particular, reflexive type activity, e.g. the corneal reflex, stapedial reflex and chewing reflex. Corticobulbar fibres descend onto the nucleus; some of these being crossed, except for those which supply the frontalis and obicularis oculi muscles which are ipsilateral. An upper motor lesion will therefore produce a contralateral paralysis of the lower facial muscles. However, these muscles will respond normally to emotional reactions. This is due to the fact that pathways mediating involuntary emotional expression do not travel through the internal capsule but are efferents from the hypothalamus and the pallidum. This explains the characteristic "mask-like" expression seen in patients with Parkinson's disease. Monrad-Krohn (1939) describes a disinhibition of emotional reaction in cases of capsular lesion. Here the patient may show signs of extreme emotional lability with alternate laughing and weeping. Higher cortical centres probably exercise a restraining influence on these subcortical behaviours. Brown (1967) discusses this phenomenon at some length.

The sensory part of the facial nerve is concerned almost entirely with taste, particularly so in the anterior two thirds of the tongue. The afferent fibres are distributed to the nucleus of the solitary tract where they are joined by fibres with similar function from the glossopharyngeal and vagus nerves. Their course from this nucleus to the sensory cortex is not fully known though most certainly it is via the thalamus.

A facial nerve paralysis (Bell's palsy) is the most common outcome of damage to the motor root. Centrally, degenerative conditions involving other bulbar nuclei will include a similar type of paralysis but there will then most likely be other signs of bulbar degeneration (progressive bulbar palsy).

The glossopharyngeal and *vagus nerves* share some common features functionally along with the *accessory nerve* and it is customary to describe them as belonging to one group.

Efferent fibres relating to special visceral functions have their origins in the *nucleus ambiguus* which is a long column of cells found in the medulla oblongata. These pathways are of considerable importance for speech production because they supply striated muscles in the larynx, pharynx, soft palate and the upper part of the oesophagus. The nucleus ambiguus receives fibres from other nuclei in the brain stem so that reflex loops in relation to vital functions like coughing, gagging, vomiting etc. exist. It also receives corticobulbar fibres.

General visceral efferent fibres which relate to the autonomic nervous system originate in the dorsal motor nucleus of the vagus and in the inferior salivatory nucleus.

The afferent component of the glossopharyngeal nerve innervates the posterior third of the tongue, adjacent parts of the oral cavity and soft palate. It is concerned with taste. Afferent components of the vagus nerve are distributed throughout the thorax and abdomen. Their main function is to do with reflex aspects of cardiovascular and respiratory activity.

The peripheral pathway of the vagus nerve merits special consideration because of its importance to speech. In particular the superior laryngeal nerve supplies an external motor branch which innervates the cricothyroid muscle and an internal branch providing sensory innervation of the larynx.

The inferior laryngeal nerve follows a slightly differing course on each side. It provides a motor supply to all laryngeal muscles (except for the cricothyroid mentioned above).

Laryngeal musculature is well endowed with mechanoreceptors as also are the cartilage joints. This underlines the importance of adequate sensory feedback to produce the appropriate balance and sequence of activity necessary for properly coordinated movement in phonation. Lesions of these nerves may have far reaching effects on resonance and phonation. Further reference will be made to these in Chapters 4 and 5.

The hypoglossal nerve is usually regarded as being purely motor. More recent studies (e.g. Sussman, 1972; Kawamura, 1970) have ascribed a sensory role to it though this has not as yet been firmly established. It innervates all the intrinsic and extrinsic muscles of the tongue, except for the palatoglossus, which is probably supplied by a branch of the vagus nerve as part of the pharyngeal complex. Any lesion of this nerve will have some effect on tongue movement though unless the trauma is severe it is likely that the tongue will respond by adopting compensatory movement.

Presetting of Cortical Mechanisms

It has been shown that prior to the actual utterance of a word there is a preparatory setting of musculature by increase of tension. Jasper, Ricci and Duane (1960) showed that changes in the electrical activity of the motor cortex did not synchronize with onset of activity but started before any activity could be detected in the muscles. This suggests that there is a preparatory setting of the motor system. Some other mechanism, a form of trigger impulse, is responsible for the translation of this preparation into initiation of activity. Wyke (1970) also refers to a pre-setting mechanism in laryngeal movement. He describes this as the result of an activity originally learned voluntarily in the course of development but assuming reflexive control thereafter. Grey Walter (1967) describes an adaptive wave of electrical discharge preceding action, the Contingent Negative Variation (CNV). This is an expectancy wave which is observed when there is a requirement to respond to a stimulus. Kornhuber and Deecke (1964) quoted by Magoun (1967) have also observed these antecedents of motor behaviour. Grey Walter (op.cit.) states that this expectancy wave is never observed in children before three years of age and that though it is not present in all normal people, it is consistently absent in disturbed or autistic children. Furthermore, it may be evoked by selective sensory stimulation in some children with speech disorders.

The foregoing descriptions have indicated some of the difficulties which present in trying to account for neurophysiological processes which underly speech. These difficulties are in part the result of the complexities of the systems which one is attempting to describe and in part the outcome of as yet insufficient knowledge. A further gap will be apparent to the reader. This is the one which lies between the intention to speak and the actual onset of the act. The previous paragraphs have described a priming mechanism but how and in what way is this initiated? Mountcastle (1980) states that before a movement can be coded into patterns of neural signals there must first be a notion, an intention of the act. This may arise in response to an external stimulus but it may equally likely be stimulated internally by thoughts or emotions. The hiatus between ideation and execution also concerns psychologists and linguists. It remains as yet unbridged.

Further reference to cranial and spinal nerve function as they relate to speech will be made in the chapters on disorders of articulation. A detailed account of speech musculature lies outside the scope of this book. For comprehensive accounts the reader is advised to read e.g. Zemlin (1968), Hardcastle (1976), Dickson and Dickson (1982).

Neurolinguistic Aspects of Speech Production 3

Overt speech is the consequence of a series of interrelated events. First there must be an intention to speak and some knowledge of the type of speech act which appropriately fits the occasion. Is the utterance for example, to be declarative, questioning or requesting? In what style must the listener be addressed? Intimate conversational or public oratorial? So that the meaning of the message may be conveyed a linguistic programme must be assembled in which lexical items are arranged in semantic and syntactic units acceptable to the particular linguistic environment. These units are in turn the outcome of patterned phonological sequences. Abstract levels of planning must then be translated into neuromuscular commands to enable the vocal tract musculature to achieve the correct configuration for the production of a sequence of sounds recognizable to the listener. Not only the listener, but also the speaker perceives the utterance through the medium of multi-sensory feedback circuits.

This outline description emphasis the dynamic nature of speech production. As such it represents a synthesis of psychological, linguistic and physiological behaviours. An analogy of chain structure is sometimes applied to speech production, but in some ways this is a misleading comparison since it suggests a straightforward linear arrangement of events each linked to the other in a predetermined sequence. Such a description is only partial and belies the complexity of the total process much of which may still be inferred only in speculative terms. Another drawback of the chain analogy is that it allows only for unidirectional activity, that is, there is provision for monitoring only *after* the utterance has taken place; any control *during* the event is precluded. Neither can it successfully allow for feedforward mechanisms whereby ongoing changes can be effected in the light of expected future occurrences.

The system by which abstract neurolinguistic planning transfers to overt speech has been the subject of much study and many theories (these were touched upon in the previous chapter).

This chapter reviews some models of speech production and in outline discusses their possible relevance to deviant conditions.

There are three broad headings which may serve as a framework for description. They are: Ideation, Execution and Control.

Ideation

Luria in 1976, wrote of "the incarnation of thought into narrative speech". Drawing upon the work of the Wurzburg school he described "thought" as "an amorphous intention without any visual or verbal form, (imageless and speechless)" (p. 4). Lashley (1951) had also earlier on been influenced by this source in the development of his ideas about what he called "The Determining Tendency". "The feeling . . . of being about to have an idea" (p. 117). The intention and formulation of the linguistic programme in effect may be seen as a confluence between cognitive aspects of psychology and neuroscience. Conditions of dementia, some confusional states and possibly certain aphasic conditions demonstrate a lack of contiguity between Idea and Execution. Understanding of the link between the two aspects remains relatively fragmentary and in the context of the present discussion on Production it is in any case somewhat tangential.

Execution

The processes which enable the planning and carrying out of spoken language are subsumed under this heading. The use of the term "spoken language" is deliberate since it is intended to draw attention to the anomalies created by a completely artificial distinction sometimes drawn between "speech" on the one hand and "language" on the other. Crystal (1981) addresses this problem and among reasons for disapprobation he notes the far from clear boundaries which demarcate motor aspects of production, referred to as *speech* and linguistic aspects traditionally referred to as *language*. Both terms will be used interchangably throughout this text.

Linguistic Programming

Neurolinguistic planning, a model of which is illustrated in Fig. 7, begins with the retrieval of semantically appropriate items with which to express the idea (Level A). Laver (1977) suggests that there is an element of redundancy in the selection process in that more items may be available than are actually utilized in the subsequent programme. This may well relate to uncertainty about which particular combination of structures best fits the expression of the idea and even indecision about its exact nature. The search for appropriate expression of particular thoughts is a familiar feeling we have all experienced. Evidence of this prolixity comes from slips of the tongue data, where it is shown that there may well have been competition between two or more semantic items either of which may have been acceptable. Laver's examples are:

"he behaved as like a fool" (like a fool + as if/though he were a fool)
"didn't bother me in the sleast" (Slightest/least) (1973, p. 135).

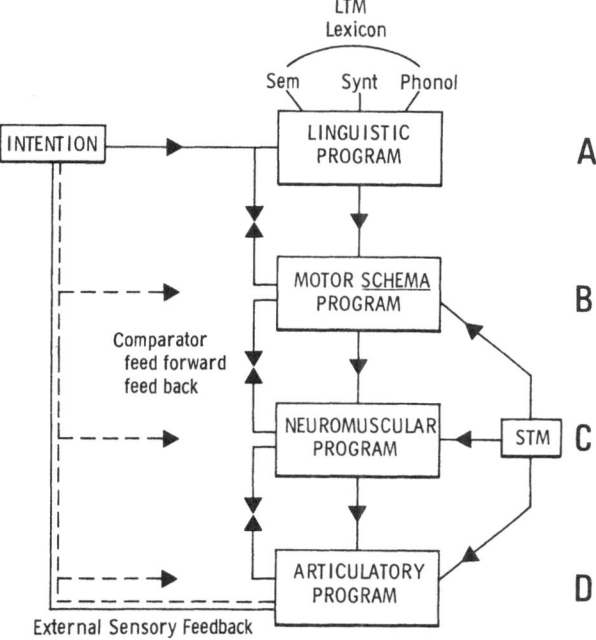

Fig. 7. Model of speech production (after J. Laver). *LTM* Long-term memory, *STM* short-term memory

Shattuck-Hufnagel (1979) describes a compatible model which posits a three part programming device wherein there is provision for serially ordered slots into which an equal number of independent segments may fit; there is a scan-copier which selects the appropriate segments for the plan, and two monitors, one of which marks the segments as they are slotted in and the other which detects and deletes any errors in the planned sequence. This model raises two questions, viz. What is the size of the units stored and what length of "speech" is preprogrammed at this level? With reference to the first question, phoneme, syllable and word have all been advanced as candidates. Evidence in favour of the phoneme as the smallest invariant unit is suggested by Liberman *et al.* (1964) but this is disputed by Kozhevnikov and Chistovich (1975) and by Fromkin (1968) who favour the syllable. In a later paper in 1977 Laver states that as yet no conclusive answer is forthcoming and suggests an expedient remedy by allowing that in a "general discussion of control aspects of the neurolinguistic system, perhaps it is sufficient to take the existence of neurolinguistic units for granted whatever their actual nature" (p. 148).

Shattuck-Hufnagel (1979) also refers to debates about units of storage. Lexical units are usually described as if they are stored in complete phonological form corresponding to surface structure. If there were no provision for the serial ordering of phonological units it would be difficult to explain error data which demonstrate misordering. She suggests that lexical items are stored in complete (abstract) form but that during production, the phonological segments must be matched one by one with appropriate slots which have been computed independently. Such a procedure would require a short term memory facility in which lexical items could be held while necessary phonological scanning copying took place. Laver's 1980 model includes provision for this type of review and correction.

The stretch of speech most likely to be preplanned is the *tone group,* Halliday (1963). This stretch of speech is, on average, of about seven or eight syllables duration with one prominent nuclear syllable on which change of pitch occurs. It is thought to correspond most nearly to the neurolinguistic planning function. It is plausible to think that a skilled activity like speech could not be carried out on a sound by sound, or even a word by word basis. Corresponding analogies in other movements, e. g. typing, piano playing have shown that sequences of movement are planned as rhythmic patterns and not as individual movements. Discussion of central nervous function in Chapter 2 already supports the view of movement as a synergism. The notion of the tone group as being the carrier of a stretch of speech is of considerable interest because as such it provides the basic framework for nonsegmental aspects of speech, i.e. rhythm, intonation, and stress. Studies of disordered speech reveal dysprosody as being one of the salient features in some conditions. If the rhythmic framework is determined at this relatively early stage in the linguistic programme this suggests the existence of two differing types of rhythmic disorder, phonological and phonetic, the former originating at an early stage in the programme and the latter being the outcome of neuromuscular dysfunction at a temporally later stage. Lenneberg (1967) has ascribed prime importance to rhythmicity not only in relation to speech but as an underpinning of much human behaviour. He compares its role with that of a pacemaker which confers a basic rhythm upon speech.

The linguistic planning stage is also noted by Lashley (1951); he refers to it as the priming of expressive units. At this covert level of planning, aggregates of words are held in readiness. Spoonerisms or contaminations he ascribes to the relative strengths of association between the different units of the utterance rather than to excitation of an excess number of competing elements. Evidence of error by association is provided by the fact that frequently the error is a word which belongs properly later on in the utterance. Speech errors are a fruitful source of example indicating planning processes, and considerable store is set in the literature by specific instances.

It is interesting to note by way of digression that the word "Spoonerism" has found its way into the English language as being synonymous with speech production errors. A fascinating essay by John Potter in 1980 attempts to disentangle fact and fable. Dr. Spooner was an Oxford academic who was born in the second half of the last century and died in 1930. Facts show that out of the hundreds of oral spoonerisms attributed to him there is substantive evidence for only about nine, though there may well have been more. One of these, quoted by Lord Russell Brain refers to an occasion when Dr. Spooner is said to have addressed him as "Brainy Russell"! There is, however, abundant evidence of his errors in writing. Potter concludes that Spooner may well have suffered from a type of dyspraxia which could have been developmental and that indeed he did evince sequencing and metathetic type disorders but that these occurred far less frequently than was attributed. His particular environment, Oxford, supplied the necessary embellishments to the true facts.

Motor Programming

The next stage in the planning programme following acceptance of the linguistic items is described by Laver (1977, 1980a) as that of abstract motor planning. This entails the preparation of schemata which reflect the requirements of the linguistic programme. The question as to what is included in the term *motor schemata* has generated much discussion and many attempts to devise models which may account for levels of storage, planning, and operation (Fig. 7, Level B).

The traditional nineteenth century view held that all necessary information for the carrying out of movement was stored in the motor cortex, and that a direct correspondence existed between excitation of specific pyramidal cells and particular neuromuscular events. This has been called the "keyboard phenomenon" because it has obvious parallels with the notion of a master controller in charge of all events. This classic view is no longer tenable in the light of present knowledge. It takes into account neither coordinating and contextual features of movement nor the complexity of sequential organization of such movement. In speech articulation, for example, production of any single sound may involve upwards of 35 muscles (Hardcastle, 1976). It must also be noted that such a single sound will vary according to its environment both in relation to neighbouring sounds and to its position within the whole sequence of utterance (allophonic variation and coarticulation). A requirement that the cerebral cortex should store so many separate commands is unrealistic. Wickelgren (1969) proposed an equally untenable storage theory, wherein he suggested the storage of context sensitive allophones each of which would slot into only one phonetic environment. If the idea of motor schemata for invariant phonemes presents a problem, in this theory it is compounded. Accounting for all possible variations this would necessitate provision for well above 100,000 items and even allowing for the extensive neuronal structure of the human brain an intolerable demand would be placed upon it in such circumstances.

The fact that a variety of muscular responses could result in the same action led Hebb in 1949 to delineate a theory which he called *motor equivalence.* This proposed that during the learning period of an activity, perceptual information from auditory, visual, tactile and proprioceptive channels is utilized to build up an internalized spatial and temporal representation of the movement, a "space coordinate system". What is stored is not a detailed plan but a schema of movement directed towards reaching a given target, MacNeilage (1970) cites the example of a good tennis player who with remarkable precision is able to hit a ball approaching him from different angles and at different speeds, and to ensure that it lands in a relatively small area of the court. To achieve this, he must have an internalized spatiotemporal representation of the whole situation in order to initiate the correct series of motor commands which will generate the necessary movements. MacNeilage considers that movement for speech is initiated in much the same manner. During development of speech the child builts up motor schemata based on the integration of afferent (sensory) and motor information. These enable him to reach articulatory targets even when compensatory action is required. Speaking through clenched teeth is an example given. The result is quite intelligible but to achieve it, there needs to be adaptive movement of the tongue and lips to accord with the limitation of mandibular excursion.

The motor equivalence view of speech production begins with the reception by the motor planner of the linguistic programme. This is then translated into a series of spatial targets which are converted into a neuromuscular programme effecting activation of the vocal tract. Laver suggests that the motor programming stage may be the source of errors in serial order of sounds. Motor equivalence therefore specifies a progression from the storage in long-term memory of a limited number of spatiotemporal coordinates which activate a much larger number of neuromuscular commands to achieve a finite articulatory state.

It will be seen that in this process the sensory system assumes a dual role. It plays a significant part in the creation of space coordinates and additionally it provides moment to moment feedback about the vocal tract. The second aspect of its role will be discussed more fully in the section describing control.

The literature on motor behaviour reflects a tendency towards increasing delegation of responsibility away from the cerebral cortex towards peripheral nervous mechanisms. The early concept of a master controller with full responsibility for all aspects of movement has given way to the idea of hierarchical control where fundamental goals are defined at high levels but their execution is dependent on successively peripheral structures until the point is reached where the desired movement is achieved. One limitation of this form of multilevel control is possible diminution of accuracy in the response because of the large number of degrees of freedom which have to be controlled in relation to the intended movement. There is also likely to be a reduction in options for response because of constraints imposed by the successive stages in the hierarchy.

Stelmach and Diggles (1982) in a review of control theories discuss the concept of *Action Theory*. This derives largely from Bernstein (1967) who proposed that movement should be divided into "functional units whose precise combination represent coordinated action" (op. cit., p. 91). This view which has been further developed by Greene (1972), Fowler (1977) and Turvey, Shaw and Mace (1979) represents a radical departure from the more traditional views of speech production programmes which assume central controls and processes. Action Theory has as its core concept the notion of coordinative structure. This is defined as "a group of muscles often spanning several joints that is constrained to act as a unit" (Turvey *et al.,* 1979, p. 563). Coordinative structures represent a compounding of reflex circuits which may be activated by a single command of either central or peripheral origin. The structures require a tuning function which selects and activates appropriate combinations of muscle units to achieve the desired action. Turvey and his colleagues suggest that the primary source of tuning is through proprioceptive circuits. Contextual information about the relationship of the body to the environment and about the properties of the environment also contribute. Easton (1978) considers that tuning may be brought about through the interaction of reflexes with each other and with signals from the cerebellum, midbrain and the cerebral cortex. A paper by Kelso and Tuller (1981) seeks to find in action theory a framework affording an explanation of verbal dyspraxia. This would appear to offer a very limited view of a perplexing condition and one which does not take into account the possible linguistic as separate from motor features.

Stelmach and Diggles remark that while pathways which could carry out tuning operations might be identified, evidence to support the notion of tuning aside from the obvious need for such a mechanism is lacking.

Aspects of the theory have a certain appeal when applied to speech production insofar as the interdependence of unitary action of a group of muscles in obviously acceptable. Coarticulation might be seen as an example where there is such synergy of movement. Kent, Carney and Severeid (1974) in a study of tongue and velar movements demonstrated the unitary nature of articulatory movement. For a given rate of speaking they showed that there was a time relationship between movement of lips, tongue and velum.

Stelmach and Diggles (1982) in their overview describe a further model of motor planning which they have termed *distributed control.* Whereas multilevel hierarchies allow for interaction between one "vertical" level and another, distributed control provides for both vertical and horizontal interaction, that is, control is dispersed throughout a number of structures which may interact to achieve the desired output. Arbib (1980, 1981) is one of the chief proponents of this theory. Essentially it represents a consensus type control rather than one of executive management. Motor schemata which are seen to correspond to muscle synergies at varying stages of refinement coordinate in control programmes to produce skilled movements. Arbib suggests neural maps as the source of input into the control. These provide information from which spatiotemporal patterns for movements may be derived. The motor controller it is suggested is layered, that is, it operates on several different levels, so that responsibility for the ultimate movement is distributed throughout many activation points. In relation to speech pathology this argues strongly against a localizationalist view (e.g. Geschwind, 1965) and supports an interactional model such as that proposed by Luria (1970).

Stelmach and Diggles exemplify Abbs' (1979) model of speech production as illustrating the theory of distributed control. He proposed a three level layered model. The primary level was the overall vocal tract configuration, the second level was concerned with specific articulatory movements necessary to meet requirements of level one (Fig. 7, Level C). The third specified individual muscles required for these articulatory movements. Compensatory adjustments are possible within elements at each level and are determined to some extent through afferent feedback. The distributed control model is seen as affording a feasible explanation of motor equivalence. It allows for compensation at subsystem level so that errors unless very close to the final output stage can be deleted or corrected before they become overt. It also provides for increasing refinement of movement from central to peripheral level thus to some extent surmounting the degrees of freedom problem posed by a hierarchical model.

The distributed control model shares some features in common with that of Laver (1980a). He separates the motor schema level from the next stage which is that of the neuromuscular command system. This division serves to underline the abstract nature of the schema and thus to endorse the ideas embodied in motor equivalence. The transition between the two stages is regarded as being particularly vulnerable to error. The early part of the motor programme is undertaken at much greater speed than the articulation stage which is relatively slow. It is possible therefore that a stacking up of tone groups in the short term memory buffer may occur. Experiments on digit recall have emphasized the fallibility of this storage mechanism. Similar information is very easily confused and in relation to speech this stage provides fertile ground for typical tongue slips. Boomer and Laver (1968) have shown that there is a marked tendency to confuse like with like. Metathesis of vowels interchange of voiceless and of voiced consonants, transfer of stressed syllables all feature as characteristic errors.

At this point the utterance becomes public (Fig. 7, Level D). Laver's model incorporates both hierarchical and heterarchical principles. At each level there is provision for both feedforward and feedback. Information is available about future and past events and there is an editing facility at each stage. Monitoring allows for correction.

Control

The previous discussion has related to the facilitation of speech. The final part of the process is concerned with control. Final is perhaps not the best choice of word since it suggests an activity coming at the end, whereas of course in fact control is operative throughout the whole programme and is in any case not linear but circular in nature.

There are essentially two major divisions in the type of control which may operate in speech production. These are open loop and closed loop. An open loop system is independent of the consequences of its output. Normally a preprogramming function is built into the model but once the operation begins there is no provision for modification until the cycle is complete. The domestic washing machine offers a good analogy. It can be preset for a number of different conditions relating to type of fabrics, colour fastness and so on, and in washing them it will carry out all necessary operations. But at no stage is it able to modify the programme to allow for different degrees of soiling of the load, differing depths of dye etc. Results can only be compared, reviewed and rectified when the wash is completed. Applied to spoken language, this would mean that an articulatory programme would be set with a prerequisite for certain configurations of the vocal tract. All commands would be prespecified and no peripheral influence would be exerted until the act was completed.

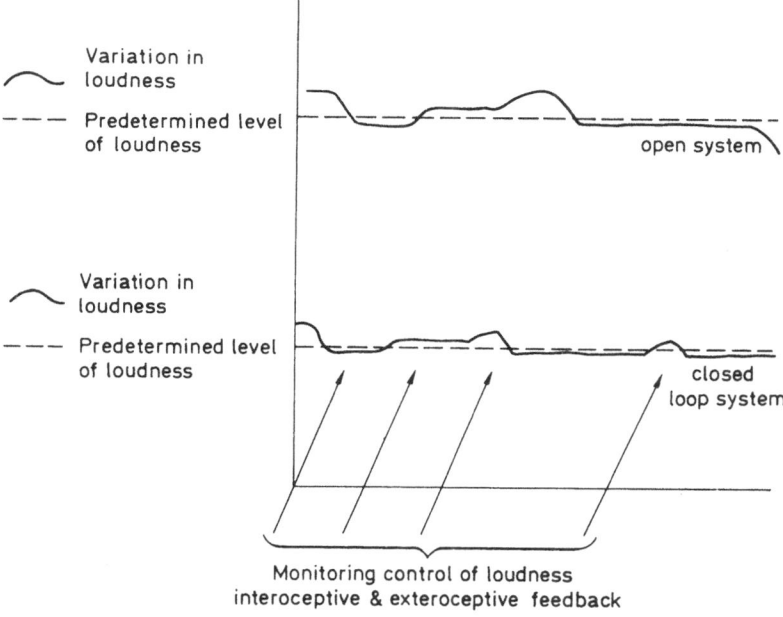

Fig. 8. Diagram showing opened and closed loop programming system

Lashley (1951) contends that this is in fact what happens. He maintains that sensory factors play only a small part in regulation and control of output once the action is learned. The speed with which many actions are performed would not allow time for sensory feedback to influence them. Some workers would dispute this on the grounds that in relation to speech the oral musculature is richly endowed with muscle spindles which provide a sufficiently rapidly acting information system to allow for feedback at least at subcortical level, Sussman (1972), Hardcastle (1976). It is therefore important to differentiate between two distinct types of feedback: sensory feedback which is relatively slow acting, and reflexogenic which is fast and which therefore probably has an intrinsic role in the control of movement.

The second type of feedback is the closed loop system. This is synonymous with a servosystem described in relation to speech by Fairbanks in 1954. A servosystem requires an effector unit, a feedback loop and a comparator device so that output may be compared with intended input, error detected and necessary corrections made.

In its pure sense the closed loop model relies entirely on sensory information generated as the result of motor activity. Any preplanning function or adjustments made during the execution of the plan do not affect it directly (indirectly of course they do since they influence the motor output). It acts upon the end result.

In practice many models of speech production incorporate features of both control systems since they are not mutually exclusive. All the motor planning models which have been described in this chapter allow for some degree of feedback either at peripheral or central level.

Types of Feedback

The classic pattern of feedback is described by Hardcastle (1976). It takes place during and after the articulatory event though it is suggested that predictive planning elements may be involved also. Two classes of feedback are described, exteroceptive and proprioceptive. Exteroceptive feedback is through auditory and tactile channels. These circuits inform the central nervous system about acoustic correlates and about changing states of contact between the articulatory organs, respectively. Both are relatively slow acting, the auditory loop being the slower. Proprioceptive feedback provides information about movement and position of the different parts of the vocal tract. A third mode of feedback may also be suggested. This is paralinguistic, it relates to listener reaction, and to the speaker's state, that is, motivation and attitude to his own utterance. Fatigue for example particularly in pathological states can exert negative influence on the degree of monitoring of speech. The factor of latency was mentioned as an objection to the influence of sensory feedback and there is certainly some divergence of view about this. Kent (1974) follows Lashley in pointing out that the delay is in the order of 200–250 ms which is much greater than the duration of a syllable. These arguments, however, refer to external feedback which takes place *after* the event. Sussman (1972), Hardcastle (1976) and Borden and Harris (1980) differentiate between external and internal feedback. The latter provides information *during* the event and acts rapidly; for example transmission of information between cerebellum and cerebral cortex takes less than 20 ms while that between thalamus and cortex is even faster. A further economy of time is suggested by Laver's model which through the notion of feedforward provides for some anticipatory priming of perceptual pathways. They are tuned to anticipate certain events and thus the detection stage can be speeded up.

MacNeilage (1970) considers the possibility of both open and closed loop circuits operating in relation to the concept of motor equivalence; the open loop would include preprogramming of the spatio-temporal target for the articulators while the closed loop would scrutinize and adjust the command in a refining operation appropriate to the particular context. The likely candidate for peripheral control would be the gamma loop though there is as yet no firm evidence of this.

Interpretation of the role of feedback in relation to speech is as with so many other aspects fraught with conflicting views. Borden (1979) in an excellent article reviews the main issues. Her discussion refers to the influence of auditory, tactile and proprioceptive feedback. Evidence from delayed auditory feedback (DAF) studies does not support the contention that auditory feedback plays a prime role once speech is established (see also Hardcastle, 1976). The same may be said for tactile feedback. About kinaesthetic feedback there is more doubt, partly on the grounds of difficulty in isolating this channel for assessment of its role. Recent work, however, discussed in the previous section of this chapter, favours the idea of internal feedback deriving from a preprogramming facility. The arguments advanced for this view however are related to established speech. In the case of developing speech external feedback channels may play a more crucial part in establishing cerebral templates of articulatory gestures. Similarly in conditions of language breakdown, strategies of therapy may need to utilize feedback as one means of reestablishing motor control.

The model of distributed control has specified the need for sharing of responsibility at successive levels of generation. This requires an intra level monitoring function provided with both feedforward and feedback facilities. Laver's (1980) model meets these requirements in terms of distribution of a responsiblity and provision for control at different levels. He distinguishes between two types of control, the first termed the planner is concerned with the editing of covert activity, the second the monitor, provides control over the overt stage of production. Laver postulates four main functions in the neuro-linguistic programme. They are:

ideation,
linguistic programming,
motor programming, and
monitoring.

These functions have been discussed in some detail. This model considers the system of control which operates throughout the entire programme. It borrows from the language of cybernetics (Wiener, 1948) and is expressed in terms of logical relationships.

The four functions (above) form part of a network of connecting *boxes*. Connections may be direct but much more frequently they are made through a series of *gates*. Some of these gates subserve the monitoring function and certain conditions are specified before input into the next box is permissable through one of the gates. Conventions for the different conditions of entry are based on Boolean logic which requires an inclusive, exclusive or partially inclusive state for operation. These conditions are termed "AND", "INCLUSIVE OR", and "EXCLUSIVE OR" (Fig. 9).

The schema for one stage, the neuromuscular conversion stage serves as an illustration of the model and is shown in Fig. 10.

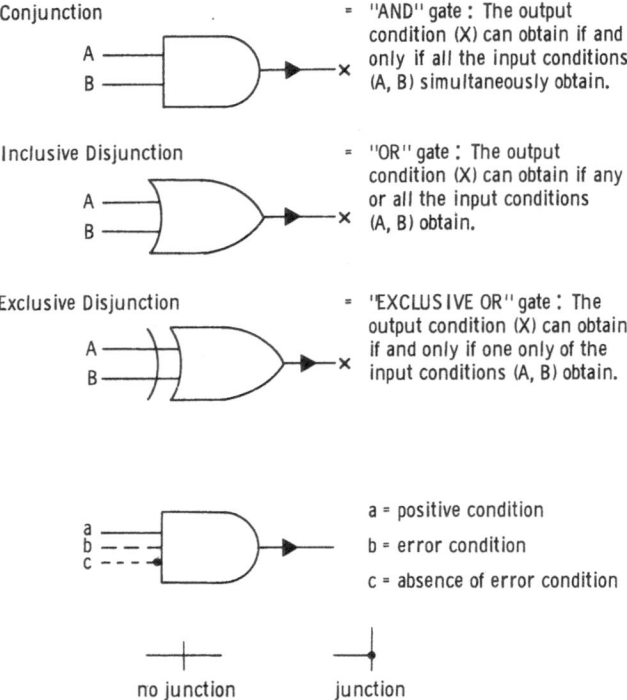

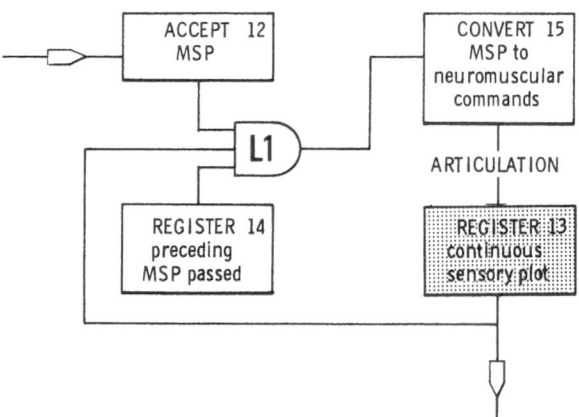

Fig. 9. Boolean Gate symbols. (Reproduced by permission of Dr. J. Laver and Academic Press)

Fig. 10. Neuromuscular conversion stage of speech production. (Reproduced by permission of Dr. J. Laver and Academic Press)

Box 12 shows that the motor schema programme (MSP) previously scrutinized and compared with the linguistic programme for goodness of fit has now been accepted. Before it can be passed for conversion to the neuro-muscular command stage its completion must be verified (Box 14). The state of the articulatory organs must also be ascertained by continuous feedback through sensory channels (Box 13). When all these conditions are satisfactorily met, Gate L1 allows passage to Box 15 and the process continues.

This particular segment illustrates just one stage in the control process. At each of the previous stages and in the final realization of the articulatory programme there is ample provision for detection and for correction. Comparator function can be carried out at each level quickly and economically through a feedforward device which utilizes preplanning of the perceptual system. A detailed description of the particular model which includes diagrammatic representation of the complete cybernetic scheme can be studied in Laver (1980).

Error data offer evidence in support of different planning levels. Nooteboom's (1981) analysis in which he reports on length of interval between error production and correction provides for an upper limit of about five syllables for phonological error and never beyond five words for lexical items. He also notes that correcting strategies which involve words frequently require a return to a point beyond where the error occurred often to the beginning of the phrase. This evidence argues in favour of a tone group type unit of planning.

Discussion in this chapter has centred on possible methods by which speech production is generated and controlled. Of necessity present knowledge has to be interspersed with speculation. But such a stance is defended by Whitaker (1971) who states that "Any model should be an attempt to integrate some good ideas with some blatantly speculative ones for the purpose of initiating further study not stultifying it." (p. 48.)

Models of speech control may be used in an attempt to identify levels of breakdown in disordered language. It has already been pointed out that one such attempt has been made in relation to verbal dyspraxia. Certainly slips of the tongue and dyspraxic errors share many features in common and these will be given more detailed consideration in the ensuing chapters. Some types of dysarthria too may provide examples of breakdown of motor equivalence. Neurological impairment may prevent the achievement of the necessary complementary state between the internalized representation and the articulatory organs. Pursuing the tennis player analogy the dysarthric patient may know exactly what configurations of muscles should be activated, but will be constrained by inability to coordinate and time the movements necessary to achieve the target.

Disorders which manifest themselves as superfluencies may well be examples of the redundancy hypothesis wherein there is defective control in the selecting and delivery of the linguistic programme. The two levels of linguistic and neuromuscular operation are in effect out of phase.

It has been noted that normal speakers make comparatively few overt errors in speaking, bearing in mind the immense complexities involved. This is taken as a testimony of the effectiveness of the covert control system. Where there is functional impairment which prevents this system operating efficiently there is likely to be a greater amount of error. This is one of the aspects to be considered in the following chapters on disorders of production.

Correlates of Dysarthria 4

Classification of dysarthria as a unitary condition is inaccurate. Peacher (1950), Grewel (1957) and Darley, Aronson and Brown (1975) all emphasize the fact that this term is a label for a *group* of disorders which share certain common features. They all stem from defined neuropathological conditions and they all combine in varying degrees of predominance, abnormalities of respiration, phonation, resonance and articulation. The majority of authors describe dysarthria as a motor disorder of speech as distinct from a disorder of language. But this may well oversimplify the issue since boundaries between motor (phonetic) and linguistic levels of production are by no means clear cut. Crystal (1981) mentions this problem when he suggests that though the primary difficulty may be phonetic, compensatory strategies used by the dysarthric speaker may give rise to syntactic and phonological anomalies. It is, however, not always readily apparent whether nonsegmental disorders originate phonetically or phonologically. Palilalia, for example, where there is a reiteration with increasing rate, of words and/or phrases is generally regarded as being a type of subcortical dysarthria, but certain features are shared with the higher order perseverations of some types of dysphasia.

The situation is further complicated because an acquired cortical dysarthria in pure form is not all that common. As very often it results from a cerebral vascular accident (CVA), some degree of dysphasic impairment may also be manifest, thus making a clear diagnosis somewhat difficult. Acquired dysarthria also bears certain similarities to verbal dyspraxia. These will be discussed further in Chapter 5.

The aim in this chapter is to consider particularly the way in which dysfunction of the supralaryngeal part of the vocal tract may result in dysarthria. By so doing it is acknowledged that this represents an incomplete picture since articulatory aspects are only one and some would suggest, a secondary part of the disorder. Because of the intimate reciprocal relationship which exists between all parts of the vocal tract, dysfunction at any one level will also influence other levels. For example, it is difficult and in any case not helpful to consider respiration without reference to phonation, phonation without reference to resonance, resonance to articulation and so on, because they are all interlinked aspects of production. A disorder at any one level will have a ripple effect throughout the entire tract. This does not mean that neuromotor impairment throughout the tract is equally disturbed; on the contrary it is well recognized that there will be varying degrees of dysfunction at different levels. But bearing in mind the previous discussion on motor equivalence, it is likely that compensatory measures will be adopted in an effort to overcome the resulting disability. An upward shift of the larynx and a backward displacement of the tongue for example are often regarded as (unsuccessful) compensatory postures to counteract hypernasal resonance.

It needs therefore to be stated that in the ensuing description, while primary concentration will be on articulatory features, these can only be discussed in the context of all levels of speech production.

This chapter is also to some extent eclectic in so far as no attempt is made to offer a comprehensive account of the dysarthrias. This task has already been fulfilled with greater competence and considerable eloquence by Darley Aronson and Brown in the report of their Mayo Clinic Study (1975). Rather the aim is to consider the dynamic features of the disorders and by drawing upon evidence from recent studies, to emphasize the contribution made by neurophysiology and neurolinguistics towards a better understanding of their nature and thus implicity towards more effective remediation.

Classification

Some broad classification is necessary as a framework for discussion. Various models have been proposed. That described by Kent (discussed in Johns, 1978) in part parallels the neurolinguistic model of speech production reviewed in the previous chapter. This organizes speech production into a series of *events* which occur at different levels of production. *Internal* events are:

> neural – this refers to the generation of programmes within the central nervous system;
> muscular – the myodynamic organization necessary for speech;
> structural – that is, the movements resulting from muscle contraction;
> aerodynamic – the changes in pressure and flow of air which take place during ongoing speech.

> *External* events are:

> acoustic – this refers to the physical properties of the sound produced viz frequency, intensity, features of articulation and temporal relationships;
> perceptual – this embodies a descriptive evaluation of speech. It relies on a subjective impression.

The Mayo Clinic Study (Darley Aronson and Brown, 1975) was the outcome of a rigorously conducted perceptual assessment of many types of dysarthria.

More recently Enderby (1980, 1983) has published an assessment which is partially perceptual and which profiles salient features of dysarthria.

Another perceptual evaluation which is more applicable to phonatory aspects has been devised by Laver (1980b). This profiles different types of phonation in terms of articulatory settings which are recorded as scalar degrees of variation from a hypothetical neutral state of the vocal tract. While being concerned primarily with a description of phonation, the profile includes assessment of tongue position, lip and jaw positions as well as respiration and laryngeal function, thus underlining the interdependence of the entire vocal tract as mentioned above.

Yorkston and Beukelman (1981) have produced an assessment which provides a measure of intelligibility and speaking rate. This and other perceptual measures will be discussed more fully in Chapter 6.

Objective measures have become increasingly available with the growth and development of electronics, and instrumentation of this type is no longer to be found only in research laboratories but is now becoming routine equipment in many speech therapy departments.

Acoustic data may be derived from spectrographic analysis which plots frequency against time. This gives information about the duration, voicing onset time, intensity, transitions and formants of sounds. Obviously considerable experience in examining normal spectrographs is necessary in order to recognize aberrant patterns.

The laryngograph (Fourcin and Abberton, 1971) yields objective information about fundamental frequency and gives a visual representation of pitch changes at laryngeal level (Fig. 11). More recently this work has been augmented by studies using xeroradiography (Berry et al., 1982). This technique depicts radiographically the interrelationship of laryngeal and supralaryngeal soft tissue structures. It provides sufficient clarity of detail to allow identification of even small muscle groups. Seventeen different parameters of the vocal tract ranging from the level of the vocal folds through to the lips are measured at rest and during phonation with resultant changes being noted. Fig. 12 shows the levels at which measurements are taken. Radiation dosage is a slight hazard in this type of investigation, though it is stated to be very small. The advent of nuclear magnetic resonance (NMR) techniques will, while providing equally comprehensive information, obviate this limitation of xeroradiography.

Aerodynamic levels can be ascertained through a variety of instrumentation which measures vital capacity, nasal and oral air flows and pressures. The Exeter nasal anenometer (Ellis and Flack, 1979) is one such type of instrument. This records changes in nasal flow during ongoing speech and is a useful means of quantifying degrees of nasal escape though this of course represents only one of the parameters contributing to hypernasal resonance (see Chapter 6, Fig. 16).

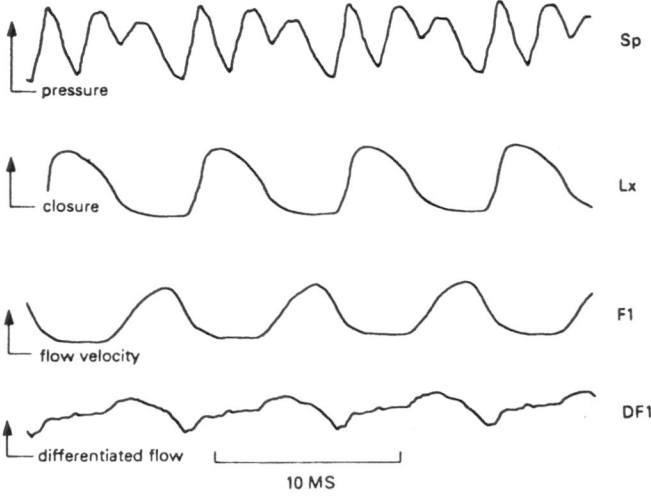

pressure — Sp

closure — Lx

flow velocity — F1

differentiated flow — DF1

10 MS

Fig. 11 a

Fig. 11. Laryngographic (Lx) wave forms demonstrating normal and abnormal phonation. In a male and female subject
a Waveforms for normal voice–normal adult male–neutral vowel. *b* Waveforms for normal voice–normal adult female–neutral vowel. *c* Waveforms for breathy voice–normal adult male–neutral vowel. *d* Waveforms for breathy voice–normal adult female–neutral vowel. (Reproduced by permission of Dr. A. J. Fourcin and American Speech and Hearing Association)

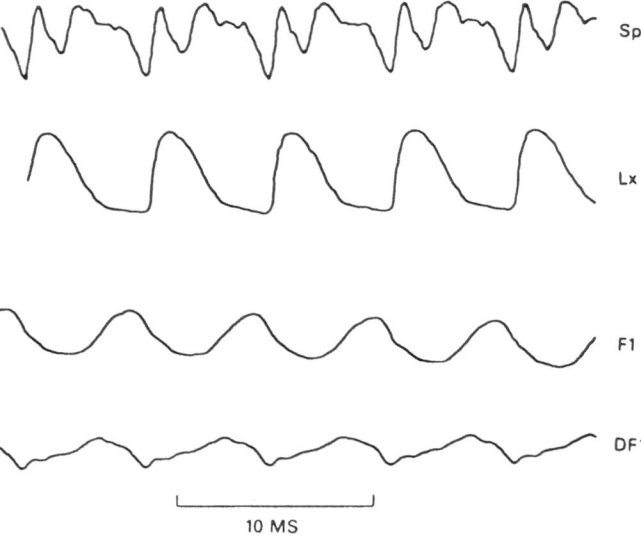

Sp

Lx

F1

DF1

10 MS

Fig. 11 b

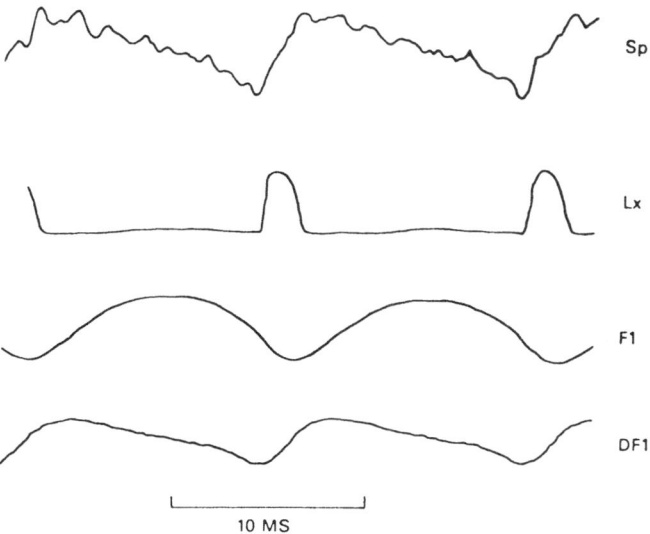

Sp

Lx

F1

DF1

10 MS

Fig. 11 c

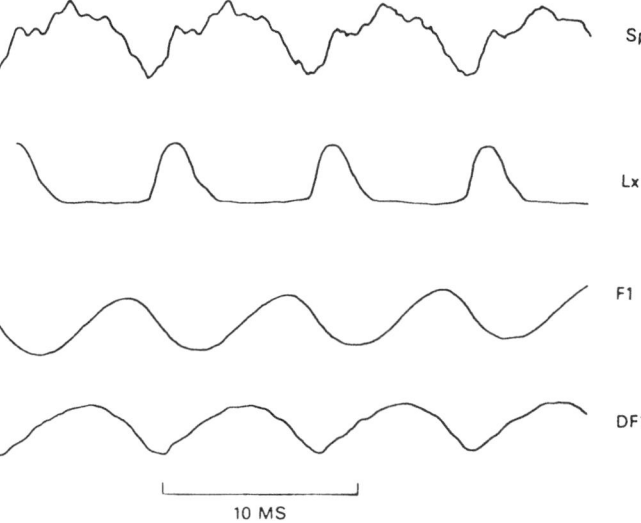

Sp

Lx

F1

DF1

10 MS

Fig. 11 d

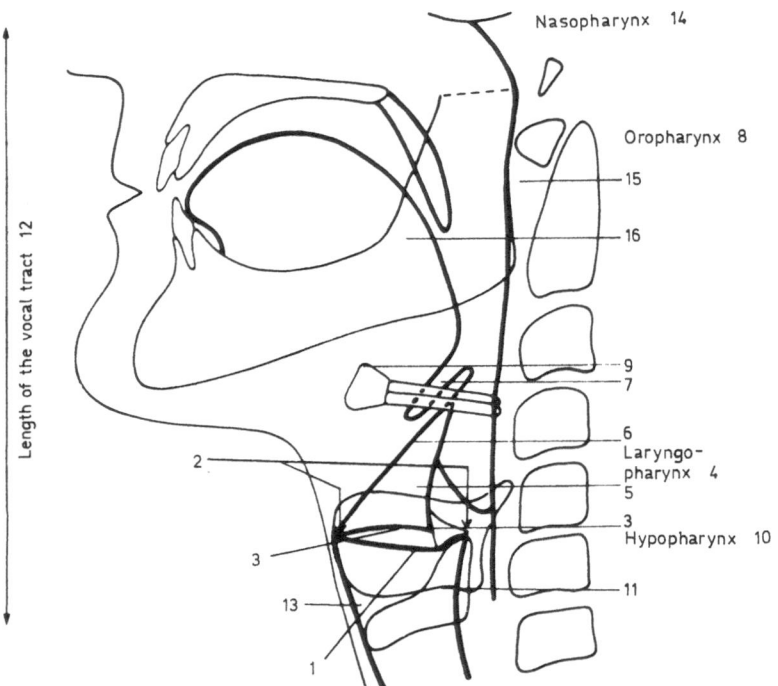

Fig. 12. Parameters of vocal tract xeroradiography. (Reproduced by permission of Dr. Frances MacCurtain and British Journal of Disorders of Communication.) Anatomical parameters: listed in order of frequency of use in analysing voice disorders. Parameter: *1* Vocal folds: anteroposterior length and position. *2* Dimension of laryngeal airway, at the level of the superior border of the vocal and arytenoid folds. Measured from the anterior extremity of the attachment of the vocal folds to the thyroid cartilage to the posterior silhouette of the cricoid cartilage. *3* Ventricular folds: superor-inferior dimension of the ventricle. *4* Laryngopharynx: anteroposterior dimension of distance between epiglottis and posterior pharyngeal wall at narrowest point. *5* Vestibule of the larynx: anteroposterior measurement at its lower border. *6* Epiglottis: distance between epiglottis tip and pharyngeal wall; height of tip; angle of epiglottis. *7* Vallecula: anteroposterior dimension. *8* Oropharynx: shape of posterior surface of tongue root in relation to pharyngeal wall: distance between tongue and wall at most retracted point. *9* Hyoid bone: the top of the front of the body, related to nearest cervical vertebra. *10* Hypopharynx: anteroposterior dimension of posterior aspect of cricoid cartilage to pharyngeal wall. *11* Level of thyroid cartilage, measured at lower border. *12* Vertical length of vocal tract, measured from spheno-occipital bone (base of skull) to inferior border of cricoid cartilage. *13* Cricothyroid vizor: measured from inferior border of anterior of thyroid cartilage to inferior border of cricoid cartilage. *14* Nasopharynx: shape of soft palate and distance from Passavant's Ridge at anterior tip of C1. *15* Retropharyngeal soft tissue: anteroposterior depth at each cervical vertebra. *16* Gesture of the tongue: e.g. tip raised; "bunching"; posterior grooving. *17* Gesture of the lips: e.g. protruding; spread

Structural events may be assessed by a number of methods. Lateral videoradiography gives a picture of ongoing movements of articulators during speech. Electropalatography (Hardcastle, 1972, 1982) provides an objective record of lingual movement as do the pellet tracking techniques which use microbeam radiography systems to record oral movements, e.g. Kiritani and his colleagues (1975). It should be mentioned that although the term "electropalatography" is widely used, in a strict etymological sense the term "electroglossography" is more correct since what is being measured is *tongue* and not *palatal* movement. Muscle action potentials, that is to say, electrical discharge which results from muscle activity can be registered through electromyography, but this is generally considered to be more accurate if intramuscular as opposed to surface electrodes are used (for recent work in this field see O'Dwyer *et al.*, 1981). See Chapter 5, Fig. 14.

Events within the central nervous system are less accessible to measurement but a certain amount of information about neural coding has been reported from extensive research carried out in Leningrad. This used patients with dyskinetic dysarthrias whose medical treatment included implants of electrodes into subcortical structures. Cerebral blood flow studies (see Wood, 1980, for review) have been used increasingly to provide information about speech processes. Of much longer standing are electroencephalographic (EEG) techniques.

There is therefore at the present time a growing amount of sophisticated equipment available which potentially can provide a much more detailed picture of factors underlying speech disorders. Obviously their use in some cases calls for a high degree of specialist knowledge and skill, but the idea of a team working together on these types of investigation is not an unrealistic expectation, particularly in many of the larger centres. A few years ago the notion of speech therapists using computers to process and store data would have seemed highly unlikely and yet this is now becoming routine practice.

Any investigation of speech disorders appears to benefit from the adoption of combined instrumental and perceptual methods. Whereas a perceptual assessment will yield an impression of the *overall* pattern of deficit, objective measurement is likely to be more valuable in providing a detailed analysis of the *components* of that pattern and thus indicating strategies for remediation.

Compatible with Kent's model is that of Netsell (1971). He describes the peripheral speech mechanism in terms of a number of functional components. As the egressive air stream travels through the vocal tract its passage is assisted or interrupted at a number of different junctures which represent control systems or valves.

Respiration is controlled by abdominal muscles, by thoracic musculature and by the diaphragm.

Phonation is controlled by the laryngeal structures.

Resonance is determined by pharyngeal and oral musculature, by the soft palate, by the tongue and by the nasal cavities.

Articulation is under the control of tongue, jaws and lips.

The features of dysarthria are regarded by Netsell as the outcome of differing degrees of defective valving at one or more of these control points so that velocity, amplitude and range of movement are altered. This classification has direct implications for remediation and extensive programmes have been developed by Rosenbek and La Pointe (1978) and by Netsell and his colleagues (1979) using this model as a basis for intervention.

Netsell's classification is therefore in a sense one concerned with peripheral aspects since it describes the overt results of covert neural dysfunction.

Darley and his fellow workers describe dysarthria in neuropathological terms, that is, they relate the differing types of speech disorder to the corresponding site of neural impairment. This leads them to describe six types of dysarthria. They are:

flaccid dysarthria associated with lower motor neurone lesions,
spastic dysarthria associated with upper motor neurone lesions,
ataxic dysarthria associated with cerebellar or cerebellar pathway lesions,
hypokinetic dysarthria associated with basal ganglia lesions,
hyperkinetic dysarthria associated with basal ganglia lesions,
mixed dysarthrias associated with lesions of multiple systems.

This terminology offers a useful means of describing the salient features of each condition and its associated speech difficulty. It is derived from an extensive study carried out at the Mayo Clinic in Rochester, Minnesota, in which speech samples were obtained from more than 200 patients who were dysarthric. The relative prominence of 38 different dimensions of deviant speech were correlated and from these, clusters of abnormal features emerged, each one revealing a pattern which broadly corresponded to the six types of dysarthria listed above. This system of analysis is thorough but extremely detailed and to be undertaken successfully requires a considerable amount of time. As it is based on perceptual judgement it is of course vulnerable to the idiosyncratic interpretation of individual users and with so many different dimensions of speech to appraise, it is extremely difficult to assign relative prominence to them. Its chief value lies in the research that underlies the final classification and this has proved to be a milestone in the recognition of different types of dysarthria.

All three classificatory systems make a significant contribution to understanding and using Mayo Clinic terminology; the following descriptions will endeavour to synthesize these models.

Spastic Dysarthria

This is usually the result of impairment or dysfunction of the cortical areas in which the pyramidal and other descending pathways originate, or of the tracts themselves. Because of the close relationship between the tracts it is rare to find a selective dysarthria as the result of damage to one component only. Although upper motor neurone damage of this type is classically associated with spasticity it is not unusual to find mixed flaccidity and spasticity and indeed immediately post lesion, the flaccid element may predominate, spasticity setting in later. Dysarthria seldom results to any marked degree of permanence from a unilateral lesion; this is because of the dual innervation of muscles concerned with articulation, the cranial nerve nuclei receiving fibres from both contra and ipsilateral fibres in the corticobulbar tract.

Spastic dysarthria may occur as a result of cerebral vascular trauma or infection and may then be associated with dysphasia.

When it is congenital it is often diagnosed as *cerebral palsy* but this is misleading since the term encompasses a whole range of developmental neuromuscular pathologies involving cortical, subcortical, cerebellar and nuclear structures.

One of the earliest neurologists to adopt this terminology in its present sense was Sigmund Freud when in 1897 he published a treatise on the subject. Prior to this the term had been used fairly indiscriminately to cover a whole range of infantile cerebral pathologies. Furthermore, Freud, true to the taxonomic tradition of neurology delineated different types of disability arising from this specific condition so anticipating later classification. Worster Drought (1974) preferred the term *congenital suprabulbar paresis* as a description of this particular type of dysarthria. He reported findings on 200 cases which ranged in severity from the incomplete syndrome where movement of only one part of the vocal tract might be impaired as for example, movement of the soft palate, through to the complete syndrome resulting in a total paresis of the oral musculature with accompanying anarthria.

Generally in spastic dysarthria all parameters of speech production are affected. Because of weakness of chest muscles, respiration is shallow and vital capacity is low so that breath support for speech is poor. Consequently, long phrases are difficult to achieve. At laryngeal level, spasticity of the vocal folds results in harshness of phonation and pitch breaks. There is little variation in intonation and because of the poor breath control, speech tends to be syllabic with equal and even stress. Thus there is little evidence of preservation of the tone group contour which it will be remembered is thought to be the unit of programming (a stretch of six or seven syllables with its nuclear stress falling towards the end of the group).

Resonance is commonly hypernasal though Darley *et al.* (1975) differentiate in degree between the hypernasality of upper motor neurone lesions and lower motor neurone disorders such as bulbar palsy where they report more marked nasality, with nasal emission of air as a frequent additional complication.

Articulation is characterized by disorders of manner rather than of placement. This reflects the inability of the articulatory organs to achieve precision and correct timing in movement from one position to another. There tends therefore to be an undershoot situation where the target is not quite reached before movement changes in preparation for the next sound position. This is marked in sounds requiring complete closure such as /p/ /b/ or /t/ /d/ when frication may often be detected in their production indicating incomplete stoppage of the air stream. Platt, Andrews and Howie (1980) and Platt, Andrews, Young and Quinn (1980) carried out a detailed study of phonological production in 50 cerebral palsied adults, 32 of whom had varying degrees of spastic dysarthria, the remainder being athetoid. Their investigations included intelligibility rating on single words and on a reading passage, a test of diadochokinesis (DDK) and a phonetic analysis of single words. Diadochokinesis refers to the ability to carry out rapid alternating movements, in this case, of the articulatory organs. The most usual means of assessing this is by repetition of the syllables (p∧/ /t∧/ /k∧/ and /p∧t∧k∧/). Measurement is either by estimating the time required to repeat the syllables a given number of times or by noting the number of repetitions achieved within a set time (Fairbanks and Spriestersbach, 1950). Platt *et al.* (1980) found similar patterns of disorder in both spastic and athetoid subjects but that the former overall performed better and were rated as being more intelligible. This still held even after taking into account the greater degree of physical handicap and the superior intelligence of the athetoid group. Sounds which proved most difficult were post alveolar fricatives /s,z/ affricates / t∫, dʒ/ and labio dental /v/. There was a significantly greater frequency of error in production of consonants occurring in the word final as against word initial position. The greatest difficulty in relation to vowels was in achieving target position for the extremes of the vowel quadrilateral [i,a,ɑ,u]. Vowel sounds [i] and [ɑ] represents extremes of oral and pharyngeal constriction, respectively.

In this study, DDK rates were found to be about half those expected of a normal population with a mean of 2.9 syllables per second. These data were based on rapid repetition of consonant, vowel syllable trains /m∧/ /p∧/ /n∧/ /t∧/ /d∧/ , /k∧/ , /g∧/ over a period of 10 seconds (Fletcher, 1972).

Platt *et al.'s* (1980) findings reflect those of earlier studies which investigated speech of cerebral palsied children (generally, athetoid and spastic types were not differentiated). Lencione (1966) found that tongue tip sounds were most frequently defective. Byrne (1959) reported the order of difficulty of production as /θ, r, ∫, s, t∫, ð/. Irwin (1956) reported similar findings and also drew attention to the greater preponderance of distortion (i.e. manner) errors over substitution (placing) errors which is also apparent throughout all these studies. Difficulties reported in most studies indicate greater involvement of sounds which call for a fine degree of neuromuscular coordination and therefore not surprisingly these prove to be a major hurdle to spastic dysarthrics.

Unfortunately the majority of reports are based on single word production and therefore do not take into account phenomena such as coarticulation, allophonic variation or nonsegmental features all of which are features of ongoing speech. Platt *et al.* (1980) also comment on the absence in their study of any consideration of the interaction between laryngeal and articulatory parameters.

Certainly a focus on one isolated section of the vocal tract is less likely to lead to a full understanding of the disability. As has been previously noted, it is the configuration of all parts of the tract which influences the end result. For example, recent xeroradiographic pictures demonstrate graphically the inter-relationship of abnormal larynx and tongue positioning in some types of phonatory disorder (MacCurtain, 1983). In summary, Platt *et al.'s* (1980) study indicates that spastic dysarthric subjects possess an intact phonemic (abstract) language system and that defective production is the result of articulatory insufficiency.

This insufficiency is often attributed to a peripheral weakness of muscles of articulation but this conclusion has been reached in the main without objective validation.

Relationship Between Speech and Non Speech Movement

Some evidence suggests that there may not be an exact correspondence between nonspeech oral movement and spontaneous speech. Miller and Hardy (1962) (cited by Lencione, 1968), basing their conclusions on photographic and radiographic materal advocate differential evaluation of speech and nonspeech activity. Hixon and Hardy (1964) substantiated this view. It is of course true that articulatory movement for speech requires a greater degree of precision and speed, but in these studies the suggestion is made that neurophysiological programmes for the two types of activity may actually be different. Love, Hagerman and Taimi (1980) studied adequacy of biting, sucking, swallowing and chewing in 60 cerebral palsied subjects whose age ranged between 3–0 and 22–11 years. All subjects were also given an articulation test, devised by Irwin (1972) which requires the repetition of several series of words. They found some evidence of a positive relationship between feeding and speech performance though this was not complete. For example, among those rated as having normal speech (N = 14), 13 demonstrated adequate feeding and 1 inadequate skill. Of those rated as having no speech (N = 19), 2 were able to carry out the feeding tasks adequately and 17 failed. Among the 17 who failed 8 showed difficulty on only one task; only 1 subject failed all five tasks (the chewing test was subdivided into chewing firm and soft substances, thus making 5 tests in all). These authors in the same study also compared abnormal oral reflexes with speech performance. These were present in 15 out of the 60 subjects. They found no systematic relationship between level of speech and the number of abnormal oral reflexes present. For example, subjects achieving a 97% score on an articulation test demonstrated 2 abnormal reflexes as did subjects with a low score of 17.9% correct articulation.

In their discussion, the authors point out the widespread practice among speech therapists of using techniques for improvement of feeding and also elimination of abnormal reflexes as necessary precursors for facilitating speech.

The somewhat inconclusive findings reported in this study indicate that while there is a trend towards interpendence of oromotor skills and speech, a concentration on therapy directed towards improvement of these may not meet with much success and indeed many therapists would endorse this view from practical experience. Other factors, such as orosensory feedback, linguistic function and intellectual status, must also be taken into consideration in remedial work. While in early prespeech stages when discrete motor programmes may not yet be established, improvement of feeding skills may serve as a satisfactory foundation, at later stages of speech development it may be more efficacious to treat the two aspects separately. It is worthwhile emphasizing the physiological specifity of speech as distinct from visceral activity since traditionally a considerable amount of time and energy has been expended in attempts to improve production by an emphasis on the adaptation of nonspeech movements, e.g. swallowing, yawning, lip smacking etc. Such oral gymnastics make little sense in neurophysiological terms. To improve speech nothing works as well as the practice of speech. A further supporting view of the specificity of articulatory programming comes from a study by Neilson and O'Dwyer published in 1981. They recorded electromyographic (EMG) data from 7 cerebrally palsied young adults 5 of whom were athetoid and 2 spastic. Readings were obtained from 16 lip, tongue and jaw muscles. These were compared with similarly obtained data from normal young adults. Their findings failed to support evidence of weakness of any of the oral musculature. Integrated EMG signals recorded during speech of the dysarthric subjects were of the same order of magnitude as those of the controls. As with the Love *et al.* (1980) study, neither did this one find evidence of persistent retained primitive reflex responses which have been attributed as being associated with dysarthria (e.g. Bobath). Primitive reflex responses could not be elicited by direct oral stimulation.

Timing and sequence of muscle activity was abnormal in speech sequences, but an interesting point was that the particular pattern of abnormality was reproduced throughout repeated utterances of the same test sentence over 50 repetitions demonstrating a consistency of error. This lends weight to the idea that a cortically induced dysarthria may be the result of faulty motor programming, in particular the failure to produce appropriate motor schemata so that correct coordinative action of muscle groups does not take place. It has been noted that the motor cortex is concerned more with planning of synergies of muscle activity rather than with individual movements. Such a view lends support to MacNeilage's theory of motor equivalence and also to the principles of Action Theory discussed in Chapter 3. Neilson and O'Dwyer suggest that disturbed motor schemata may come about as the result of deficient transmission in descending pathways. Any impairment of sensorimotor integration processes would prevent the formulation of appropriate motor commands. One possibility is that there could be an interruption in the flow of nervous impulses between the cerebellum and the basal ganglia before they reach the motor cortex.

Benson (1962) reporting on a 13 month old child with dysphagia, described the soft palate as flaccid and discoordinated in movement though EMG readings recorded normal activity. It was concluded that this was an example of a minimal suprabulbar palsy caused by perinatal anoxia. The dysphagia improved after stimulation of oral musculature through feeding, thus possibly indicating that at this very early stage motor schemata are not firmly established and are amenable to change possibly by influence from exteroceptive feedback.

To summarize, spastic dysarthria affects the entire vocal tract at respiratory, phonatory, resonatory and articulatory levels. Articulatory disorders appear to indicate that the linguistic programming stage may be unimpaired but that there may be a failure in the laying down of motor schemata to effect synergies of movement necessary for coordinated articulation. These schemata are deficient in relation to temporal and spatial features and this is manifest overtly by slowing down and laboured speech which is defective more in precision rather than in gross error of placement.

Dyskinetic Dysarthria

Darley, Aronson and Brown (1975) differentiate between quick and slow hyperkinetic syndromes though they emphasize that this is a matter of relativity and suggest that a qualifying adjective such as *predominantly* may be a useful addition to the term. Among the quick types are the tics, myoclonic and the choreiform disorders. Slow hyperkinesias are manifest as athetosis and dystonia. There is now a general trend towards the use of generic terminology of both types as Dyskinetic dysarthrias

Dysarthria arising from any of these conditions embodies its definition as a movement disorder. Speech is interrupted by rhythmic, extraneous movement spasms which interfere drastically with its smooth flow. This appears to be the result of a disinhibition of movement whereby the regulatory influence of the cerebellum and basal ganglia acting through the thalamus is impaired so that there is inadequate control over the excess overflow of movement generated by the cortex. Bell (1968) in a report on results of cryogenic surgery for Parkinson's disease in which the site of lesion was the ventrolateral thalamic nucleus found that postoperatively there was a marked and lasting deterioration in speech though the type of dysarthria is not described in detail. He also refers to a diminution in volume of voice.

Prosody is the most prominently affected aspect of production in hyperkinetic dysarthrias. The constant disruption of speech by involuntary movement has a marked effect on rate and rhythm. The Mayo Clinic Study rated abnormal pause, variable rate and monopitch as next in rank order of prevalence after imprecise consonants.

Tardive dyskinesia is classified among these dysarthrias. This is a potentially irreversible movement disorder which presents with choreoathetoid movements of limbs and oral structures. It is commonly induced by prolonged administration of neuroleptic drugs such as phenothiazine. Portnoy (1979) notes that dysarthric speech is one of the earliest signs. It is characterized by prosodic abnormality which includes a flat pattern of intonation with little rise and fall and a corresponding monotony of loudness. Articulatory realization is irregular as a result of uncontrolled change in movement of the organs of articulation.

The present author together with a colleague, Elizabeth McGuirk, analysed the speech of 12 male patients diagnosed as chronic schizophrenics who were attending a psychiatric hospital. All had been treated with phenothiazine over varying periods of time. The following parameters were assessed from an audiotape recording of standard interview procedures between the psychiatrist and patient:

articulation,
prosody,
phonation, and resonance.

Deviances were observed in all but one of the subjects. In relation to:

Articulation: deletion of sound segments and of syllables were the most common errors which gave an overall impression of slurred speech. There were some phonological substitutions but these could have been dialectal, e.g. three / θri → tri/.

Prosody: 6 subjects showed abnormal features. 3 had repetitive falling patterns of intonation. 2 had equal and even stress with no marked nuclear stress in tone units. 4 subjects demonstrated marked pausing in their responses. These were unfilled. 2 subjects had abnormally fast rates of production. Taking an average count of 6 ± 1 syllabes/second these averaged 8 and 9 syllables/second. A third subject superficially appeared to come into this category, but analysis revealed extraneous and meaningless noises interspersed with his responses.

Phonation: 5 subjects had some abnormality of phonation and/or resonance. 2 used a consistently high pitch with narrow rise and fall. 1 had mixed modal and falsetto phonation. 1 had hoarseness with creaky phonation. 1 had diminished volume and some hypernasality.

All the subjects were given the Porch Test of Communicative Ability (PICA) to ascertain whether other levels of language were affected. Tasks requiring precise gesture were poorly performed and there was evidence of some extraneous movement of limbs.

It was not possible to extrapolate from this study any definitive causal relationship between the speech disorders and medication. Variables which were not controlled were: previous history which included alcoholism in at least two cases, and the abnormal state of affect directly relating to the illness. The falling intonation pattern and the abnormal pauses were possibly indicative of this.

Athetosis

As with spastic cerebral palsy this condition is often congenital. It is frequently associated with spasticity producing a mixed type of disability. Hearing loss is also a commonly associated condition and in these cases there is usually evidence of damage to basal ganglia and to the eighth cranial nerve. Perinatal anoxia, Rh. incompatibility and kernicterus have been cited as causative factors.

Hearing loss may be peripheral or central, more frequently the latter, and it may differentially affect high frequencies or the whole range, leading to profound deafness.

Fisch (1964) suggested that the poor auditory acuity might be compounded by what he termed "poor listening". Listening he states requires a neuro-sensory, neuromuscular and automatic involuntary response. The neurosensory component is attentional, that is to say it entails the ability to select meaningful auditory stimuli from the acoustic environment and to inhibit those which are irrelevant. Anatomically this function relates to the reticular system.

Neuromuscular requirements include the physical set, for example holding the head in a position best suited to locate sound.

Automatic involuntary reaction to sound involves changes in breathing patterns.

Kent and Netsell (1978) carried out a cinefluorographic study of oral movement in five athetoid subjects age range 12–26. Three of the five wore a palatal lift to aid velopharyngeal closure and one had undergone pharyngeal flap surgery. They observed marked reduction of tongue movement in an antero-posterior direction. This finding is confirmed by Platt and his colleagues' (1980) phonetic data which indicated that their subjects had difficulty in achieving extremes of vowel position. Velar movement was minimal. In contrast the mandible and the hyoid bone had a wider range of movement than normal, assumed to be perhaps a result of compensatory action.

Sequence of movements of lip, tongue and velum was erratic. In the sequences [əbʌ] [ətʌ], for example, in the case of the normal speaker the velum effects contact with the posterior pharyngeal wall *before* the utterance begins. The athetoid subjects did not achieve closure until the onset of the stop closure phase; thus there was nasal emission, through the delayed operation of the velopharyngeal sphincter. In some cases this was delayed until *after* lip or tongue closure had been made.

Utterance of the sentence "Please buy me that cute little dog" revealed excessive opening both in frequency and range of the velopharyngeal port; there was also premature opening in the production of a non-nasal sound so that it tended to become nasalized.

Discussing the overall timing and coordinating abnormality, the authors comment that this might reflect a failure of reciprocal relationship between agonist and antagonist muscle groups.

Another explanation is that excessive contraction of the prime movers might result in difficulty in grading onset and offset of movement.

A third possibility considered is that the exaggerated and erratic movement might be the result of a disturbance or (if congenital) a failure of proprioceptive feedback. Kent and Netsell also suggest that the abnormalities might stem from poorly developed motor schemata.

In Chapter 3 the relative roles of feedback and feedforward processes were discussed. The congenital athetoid has less favourable opportunity for acquisition of motor control since he lacks the conditions for the development of adequate motor schemata. He is also denied the opportunity for comparing actual with intended performance. It is suggested that some of these difficulties might be ameliorated by the use of biofeedback techniques to provide the monitoring facility which does not occur naturally.

Studies reflect some variation as to the similarities and differences between types of articulation disorder in athetoid and spastic cerebral palsy. Platt *et al.* (1980) in their study which comprized 32 spastic and 18 athetoid subjects did not find marked differences in the two groups; those which occurred related more to severity rather than to type of defect. They found spastics to be more intelligible than the athetoids. Some comparative studies do not allow for severity of condition but this study took into account the differing degrees of disability between the two groups and also the superior intelligence of the athetoid subjects. As in the Kent and Netsell (1978) study it is suggested that certain abnormal patterns of movement arose as a result of compensatory measures so that, for example, lips and jaw might assist in production of a lingual sound which it would be difficult for the tongue to produce in the normal way. Analysis of the data does not reveal a comparable degree of nasal defects as in the Kent and Netsell study but this may be simply a bias in choice of subjects since all of the latter's subjects had known velopharyngeal incompetence. Platt *et al.'s* subjects did show a high percentage of voicing/devoicing errors. If one considers motor planning as having linked spatio-temporal properties, then erratic timing in the adduction and abduction of the vocal folds would account for this. This feature has been observed also in dyspraxic patients and is then generally attributed to a deficit of motor planning (Freeman, Sands and Harris, 1978).

Hypokinetic Dysarthria

The substantia nigra is heavily pigmented with melanin. Dopamine is normally present in the cells containing this pigment and it is thought that in some complex way the two are metabolically related. Barr (1979) suggests that melanin may be an inert by-product of biochemical action in the substantia nigra to produce dopamine. There is a marked diminution or even absence of dopamine in the pigmented cells of patients with Parkinson's disease. The administration of a dopa-related chemical L-dopa produces to some extent the required regulatory action on excessive muscle tone and is now a widely used form of chemotherapy (see below).

Parkinson's disease represents the most commonly occurring form of this "basal ganglia" syndrome A deficiency of the neural transmitter Dopamine is cited as the cause. Dopamine acts as an inhibitor in contrast to acetylcholine which is facilitatory. Historically basal ganglia pathology has been associated with impairment of motor speech only, but this is probably an oversimplified view of cerebral function. More recently language has come to be regarded as the outcome of multiple centre participation at both cortical and subcortical levels. Kornhuber (1977) and quoted in Brunner, Kornhuber, Seemüller, Suger and Wallesch (1982) describes the role of the basal ganglia as a "program generator for language with essential participation in the organization of higher mental functions" (p. 282). The same paper discusses resultant language deficits in a series of patients with different combinations of lesions: pre-Rolandic, post-Rolandic and basal ganglia. These workers found that a lesion of Broca's area (i.e. pre-Rolandic) alone, produced only transient linguistic disorder but when there was an accompanying lesion in the basal ganglia – notably in the lenticular nucleus, dysphasia was severe and long lasting. Similarly a lesion in Wernicke's area alone, resulted in a marked dysphasia which was greatly exacerbated when there was also involvement of the subcortical nuclei. While, therefore, a disorder of speech production may represent the predominating difficulty in basal ganglia pathology, the possibility of the presence of "higher cortical linguistic disturbances" should also be considered. In Parkinsonism there may be on the one hand a marked reduction in speed and range of movement or on the other the condition may produce uncontrolled acceleration of movement. There is also rigidity.

The disease arises from a number of causes. Darley, Aronson and Brown make reference to the post-encephalitic type which was prevalent as a sequel of the virus influenza which reached epidemic incidence following the 1914–1918 war. Arteriosclerotic conditions affecting brain tissue may be the most common cause in the elderly, but head trauma and toxicity have also been cited as causative factors. Quite often, however, the aetiology is unknown. Medical treatment included in early days, administration of belladonna. This gave way to stereotaxic surgery which produced variable results particularly in relation to speech. Allan, Turner and Gadea Cirea (1966) reported on speech following surgery for 118 parkinsonian patients.

Three parameters of production were assessed: volume, articulation and function (function here refers to signs of aphasia). These were assessed pre- and postoperatively.

As might have been predicted there was a considerably more marked deterioration in speech in cases where the lesion had been made on the left side.

Subjects who had undergone left or bilateral/multiple surgery showed marked diminution in volume: 67% and 56%, respectively.

Articulation showed a similar pattern of deleterious change, 54% and 66% of subjects deteriorated immediately postoperatively. It was observed that a number of patients (39%) who had normal articulation preoperatively developed dysarthria after surgery.

It appeared that there was a greater likelihood of dysarthria as a sequal of multiple operation where right lesion followed left than in the reverse case.

No details are given about the articulatory assessments carried out in this study, therefore it is not possible to ascertain whether it was predominantly segmental or whether and if so to what degree nonsegmental properties were impaired.

All the assessments took place very soon after surgery round about the third day. No long-term follow up has been reported.

Function as related to aphasic impairment indicates that this was comparatively rare and where it occurred following left sided lesions was transient.

The site of lesion varies as does the technique employed. Critchley (1981) in a comprehensive review paper states that a double ipsilateral lesion of thalamo capsular and pallido capsular region is standard. Tremor is alleviated by the thalamic lesion and rigidity by the pallidum lesion. Thermocoagulation, cryogenic and chemical methods have all been used. Surgery is usually carried out under light anaesthetic so that with a conscious patient any changes in speech may be monitored and ongoing modification can then be made in siting the lesion. It must be stated, however, that with reference to speech, surgery on the whole has a deleterious effect. This is particularly so if speech was poor prior to surgery; it may then become very much more disordered.

Reports on speech status following chemotherapy are equivocal. Nakano, Zubick and Tyler (1973) carried out a double-blind study on 17 parkinsonian subjects aged between 42 and 74. Different types of medication which included levodopa and also no drug therapy were administered over a period. Results indicated a significant improvement in speech intelligibility as a result of levodopa therapy in 15 out of 17 subjects. The remaining two developed dyskinesias with associated deterioration of speech. Other studies, however, have shown minimal improvement in speech following medication (e.g. Leanderson, Myerson and Persson, 1971).

In the long term the improvement may not be sustained and prolonged dosage of levodopa may in fact induce further dyskinesias thus exacerbating the dysarthria. These may take the form of involuntary tongue and lip movements, abnormal respiratory activity all affecting phonation, resonance and articulation. Critchley (1981) comments on the differential effect of drug related doses of levodopa. In some cases abstention from the daily dosage produces marked improvement in speech but deterioration in locomotor ability, thus underlining the fact that different motor schemata probably are involved in speech and locomotion. Anticholinergic drugs are also sometimes administered but reported beneficial effects are few. A study carried out by Millac et al. in 1970 on the effect of Amantadine on speech indicated little improvement. Withdrawal of anticholinergic drugs may result in a marked exacerbation of the symptoms.

Koller (1983) studied dysfluency symptoms in six parkinsonian patients. He reported that levodopa therapy had no improvement effect on speech, though one patient had responded well to pergolide mesylate therapy. This facilitates the release of dopamine from the receptors. These variable results give rise to the interesting speculation that a neurotransmitter other than dopamine may influence speech movement.

The Mayo Study rated prosodic features as being most markedly affected in Parkinson's disease. In rank order these were listed as monopitch, reduced stress, monoloudness, with inappropriate silences and short rushes also high on the list of deviances. These are presumably phonetic descriptions.

One of the perplexing features demonstrated by Parkinson patients is the condition known as Kinesia paradoxica. This relates to the variability of response. Under controlled conditions such as repetition of single words or short phrases the patient may be completely intelligible whereas spontaneous speech will show all the classical signs of difficulty of inception, acceleration and deterioration in volume of speech.

Crystal (1981) presents a schema for evaluating prosodic disability in relation in intonation. He makes the point that it is important to differentiate between phonetic and phonological features. A phonetically based disorder he terms dysprosody, a phonological disorder prosodic disability. The former are the result of a general motor disability and will be apparent regardless of the language spoken. Prosodic disability, however, is allied to the phonology of the language spoken and the abnormalities may not readily be applicable to other languages. The distinction is, however, not always apparent in complex disorders like hypokinetic dysarthria where there may be a mix of both phonological and phonetic disorder.

Crystal suggests three parameters along which nonsegmental properties of intonation may be evaluated. There are: tone units, tonicity and tone.

Tone units refers to the hypothesized stretch of speech which forms the basic programming unit. The proportion of these should be observed. Too few gives the impression of unpunctuated speech, while too many renders it slow and stilted (cf. scanning speech of ataxic dysarthria).

Tonicity refers to the position of maximal prominence (stress) on a syllable. Two main ways in which this may be abnormal are by conferring tonicity on inappropriate items and by not stressing items which would normally be tonic. The third property *tone* refers to the range and direction of pitch within the system. Discussing abnormalities of pitch, Crystal lists:

flattening conferring a level tone on the utterance;
widening in which the whole of the voice range is used in an erratic and semantically inappropriate fashion, cf. ataxic dysarthria;
diminishing this represents a progressive narrowing of pitch range as the utterance proceeds;
laryngeal the abnormal function of the larynx constrains phonation is that the nuclear tone may be altered by characteristics such as whisperiness, creak, harshness, etc. (Laver, 1980b).

Mrs. E.S., aged 58 years, who has had idiopathic Parkinson's disease for 30 years, illustrates this condition well. Her articulation is poor, but this is most specifically related to her difficulty in controlling rate and range of movement in ongoing speech. On a word by word basis she is intelligible but spontaneous speech shows wild fluctuations of pitch and rate. It seems as if deprived of the harnessing framework of prosody other levels of speech production are also drastically affected. In Crystal's terms her speech might be described in the following manner:

On imitation she is able to reproduce appropriate contours with nuclear stress and normal pitch range. Spontaneous speech, however, while initially intelligible quickly deteriorates because of dissolution of nonsegmental features. Separate tone units become indistinguishable and as a corollary, tonicity is absent. Tone while tending towards repetitive flattening occasionally veers up and down inappropriately as illustrated in the utterance:

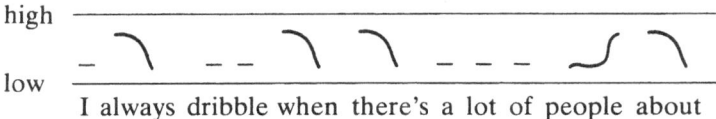

I always dribble when there's a lot of people about

Rate shows characteristic acceleration so that articulation quickly deteriorates. Arrows indicate abnormal shift of pirch, in this case upwards.

Acceleration in rate of utterance and lack of rhythmicity are quoted in most of the studies describing hypokinetic dysarthria. Kreul (1972) examined diadochokinetic rates in three groups of patients: healthy young adults

N = 45, mean age 22; healthy elderly people N = 22, mean age 70 years and 23 postsurgical Parkinson patients, mean age 56 years. He also measured laryngeal and respiratory control. Subjects were required to carry out rapid repetitions of syllables /p ʌ / /t ʌ / / and /k ʌ /, an interrupted vowel /i/ and vowel transition /u−i/. A two-second sample was counted for number of repetitions in each group. Ability to sustain prolonged vowels was timed and the study also included measurements of reading rate.

Rate of repetition of syllables was not a distinguishing feature between the Parkinson and control subjects, but there was a difference between the groups in the vowel interruption and transition tasks.

The data on syllable repetition contrasts with Canter's report published in 1965 when he found that the group overall demonstrated significant impairment in repetition tasks and furthermore that in some cases it proved impossible to evaluate because of "articulatory freeze" during which it was difficult to distinguish discrete sounds. He reported a high correlation between impairment of lip, tip of tongue and back of tongue movement which he took to be indicative of the importance of coordinative function in oral musculature. Canter's subjects were required to sustain the repetition over a 30 second period as against the 2 second time of Kreul's subjects. This could be a relevant factor in accounting for different results since decrement over a lengthening period of utterance is a characteristic feature of this type of dysarthria.

Acceleration and weakness were two features studied by Netsell, Daniel and Celesia (1975) in an electromyographic study of 22 parkinson subjects. All cases were at least 10 years post onset, all were being treated by anti-parkinsonian medication and additionally some had undergone unilateral or bilateral thalamic surgery. The findings of this study are interesting in that EMG readings confirm a subjective impression of acceleration on repetition of syllable /pɑ/ which was accompanied by a deterioration of lip contact for the /p/ sound. Increase in rate was significant. Subjects were asked to aim for a target of about 4 syllables per second, but one produced a rate of more than 13 syllables per second. This exceeds a normal top rate of 8−9 per second. The authors see this as evidence of loss of direct control over neuromuscular activity. But they caution against too ready a comparison between this type of accelerated speech and festinating gait since the two were not always associated in this study. This is also demonstrated by different reactions to dopaminergic medication as described above.

Increase in loudness produced a slowing down of rate with more control over articulatory movement. Lenneberg (1967) describes a superfluent patient though the pathology is not stated. His speech gave the impression of gathering momentum until it finally became completely out of control. Analysis revealed, however, that the rate of articulatory movements actually relevant to the utterance was in fact slow, but that these were interspersed with other inappropriate, irrelevant movements. This state Lenneberg ascribed to a disinhibition of the speech pacemaker which exercises a controlling rhythmical influence on output of speech. The subject was incidentally able to control rate in singing well known songs.

Netsell and his colleagues (1975) were interested in the apparently paradoxical situation of both speeded up and slowed down speech as characteristics of hypokinetic dysarthria. The slowing down they ascribed to rigidity of musculature which is usually diminished as an effect of drug therapy. A speculative and controversial explanation is offered by their reference to Hassler's work which posits two disparate neural circuits connecting the cerebral cortex, basal ganglia and cerebellum. Differential involvement of these circuits results in different types of impairment. Rigidity and slowness of speech is the outcome of anterior circuit involvement while posterior circuit damage produces accelerated speech and/or tremor (for discussion challenging Hassler's theory see Samra et al., 1969). In practice it is often the case that both aspects are present in varying degrees.

Netsell et al. (1975) found no indication of peripheral muscular weakness, but diminished muscle action potentials were interpreted as deficits in the neuromuscular command signals. The origin of impaired movement is therefore central and in neurolinguistic terms probably occurs between motor schema and neuromuscular programming levels.

Another type of acceleration disorder is a comparatively rare perseverative condition called *palilalia*. This takes the form of increasingly fast reiteration of utterances with diminishing loudness and reduced intelligibility. It has been described in a number of studies; in 1975 by Boller, Albert and Denes as a familial condition and more recently in a single case study by La Pointe and Horner (1981). Though there are obvious similarities to stuttering behaviour this repetitive utterance appears to be confined mostly to words and phrases. However, in some respects it closely resembles the dysfluencies of dysphasia and dyspraxia so that a differential diagnosis may not be easy. La Pointe's and Horner's subject was a 29 year-old male whose palilalia was of 4 year's standing. An unconfirmed aetiology was barbiturate addiction. A sample recording totalling 5,489 words was obtained in various task situations; of these 38% of the utterances were reiterative. In a task requiring a paraphrase of the proverb "Look before you leap" no less than 52 successive repetitions were recorded. The more automatic the task the less frequent was the repetition, and in counting and serial speech it was virtually absent. This study revealed eight different types of repetition, these being of one word, various forms of phrase, sentence and syllabic types. Word level was most susceptible and verbs were the most frequently reiterated followed by adjectives and nouns. Words with consonant cluster, e.g. /kl-, pr-/ in initial position were particularly vulnerable.

This condition which is associated with basal ganglia pathology raises interesting and perplexing questions about the part played by subcortical structures in the facilitation and inhibition of speech. It suggests a failure of inhibitory mechanisms which may correspond to perseverative choreiform and ballistic movements associated with basal ganglia lesions. Once a string of utterance (? the tone group) is initiated, inhibitory action is necessary for damping it to effect excitation of the next utterance. In palilalia the inhibitory action is not effective and like a needle stuck in a record groove the utterance is repeated over and over again until inertia sets in. The failure in inception of speech which characterizes some types of parkinsonistic disorder is probably another facet of this type of difficulty; in this case inhibitory factors overrule facilitating production.

The disfluency associated with Parkinson's disease has frequently been compared with stuttering behaviour and in some respects it bears a close resemblance to the hesitations and blocks which are a feature of stuttering. Koller (1983) describes six Parkinson patients in whom such symptoms were present. In all cases speech was characterized by repetitions and prolongations on both content and function words. Blocks occurred principally in syllable initial and medial position, rarely in final position. Spontaneous speech was markedly more affected than serial speech. These symptoms were noted very early on in the disease. Immediate repetition produced improvement; in this respect the disfluency differs from that of developmental stuttering where this effect occurs less commonly.

A detailed study of articulatory abnormalities in Parkinson's disease has been carried out by Logemann and Fisher (1981). They used the sentence analysis section of their test as a basis for sampling. This has the advantage of providing examples of ongoing speech so that there is access to information about possible planning strategies. There were 200 patients in the study and of these 90 (45%) had some articulatory error. Analysis revealed that:

Stop consonants tended to become fricative while placing and voicing remained appropriate: $[k \rightarrow X]$, $[g \rightarrow \gamma]$, $[p \rightarrow \Phi]$, $[b \rightarrow \beta]$.

Fricative consonants were reduced in sharpness, that is to say there was reduced turbulence and there was increased degree of opening through which the breath stream passed. The diacritic ^{T} is used to denote lower tongue position, so that: $[s \rightarrow s^T]$, $[z \rightarrow z^T]$.

Labiodental fricatives /f/ and /v/ became bilabialized and friction was reduced resulting in change in place and manner.

These errors reflect inadequate tongue movement and labial closure so that valving at the appropriate point was not possible. As in the Netsell study, Logemann and Fisher emphasize that this typical "undershoot" misarticulation is not caused by peripheral weakness but is central (neurogenic) in origin.

Ataxic Dysarthria

First impressions of this type of disorder are of a scanning monotonous sing song type of delivery. Intonational contours with appropriate nuclear stress (tonicity) are absent so that speech like unpunctuated writing may be virtually unintelligible. The Mayo school included this aspect under the heading of excess and equal stress which was ranked second in degree of severity, in monopitch, monoloudness and slow rate (eighth, ninth and tenth, respectively). Although slow rate received a low rating the authors observe that the cerebellar group is only exceeded in slowness by the amyotrophic lateral sclerosis and pseudobulbar palsy groups.

Ataxic dysarthria is the result of damage to the cerebellum. This may arise from neoplasms, toxicity, vascular disease or trauma (alcohol toxicity is a common cause). Sometimes cerebellar dysfunction is part of a widespread generalized disease process as in multiple sclerosis or Friedreich's ataxia.

Clinical signs of cerebellar pathology may include hypotonia, dysmetria (the impairment of distance judgement as shown in past pointing), incoordination of movement, difficulty in inception and inhibition of movement, ataxia of gait and intention tremor.

The analysis of acoustic correlates of ataxic dysarthria has been the subject of detailed studies over a number of years by workers at Wisconsin University, Madison (e.g. Kent and Netsell, 1975; Kent, Netsell and Abbs, 1979). Much of the following description is based on their findings.

The 1979 report is a description of data obtained from five ataxic dysarthric patients representing successive degrees of severity. Measurements were derived from recorded repetition of six sentences, repetition of consonant-vowel-consonant (CVC) syllables which included a range of vowels, repetition of syllable trains /pɑ/, counting 1–20 and a series of base words to which suffixes were added to produce two and three syllable utterances, e.g. *work, workman, workmanship*. By means of spectrographic analysis they were able to obtain data about formant frequencies, durational and timing features which were contributory to the characteristic dysprosody of the condition.

The most marked and consistent abnormalities were associated with duration and timing. The ataxic subjects when compared with normal controls all showed some degree of lengthening of word segments. The amount seemed to be in direct relation to the severity of the dysarthria. Overall duration of words was considerably greater, for example, 854 ms for the most severe dysarthric to produce the word *strikes* compared with a normal group mean of 389 ms.

Lax vowels were prolonged and in some cases approached duration of tense vowels so that [ʊ → u], [I → i].

In the task requiring addition of syllables to a base word, the duration of the stem is normally adjusted as the number of syllables increases. The ataxic patients showed inconsistency in this; in fact, in some instances far from reduction of stem word duration it was actually lengthened.

Spectrographic data from conversation stretches showed a striking regularity of syllabic production with distinct segregation of segments. This is what is perceptually recognized as the scanning element of the speech disorder. Also shown were two consistent features of the f_0 contour; these were a flat lower contour with a top pattern showing a fall on each syllable. This gives a monotonous character to the utterance and Crystal also describes this particular repetitive pattern of pitch fall in relation to certain types of neurological disorder (1981). It is very typical of ataxic dysarthria, but this may be interspersed with quite erratic swoops in frequency change. The inconsistency and unpredictability of the pitch changes was noted by Kent and Netsell (1975) in a single case study which included cineradiographic measurement of articulatory positions. This demonstrated variability in achieving articulatory targets. Sometimes there was a failure to make contact as in *be-an* for *began*, sometimes contact was prolonged as for example in lengthening of vowels and sometimes it was incomplete as when stops had fricative features.

Grunwell and Huskins (1979) reporting on a case of ataxic dysarthria note essentially the same deviances as those described above. However, they thought that the failure to signal meaningful intonational contrasts was of minor significance in the totality of the disorder. What they did consider to be a paramount feature was the abnormal rhythmic structure (equal and even stress) which greatly impaired intelligibility.

Bearing in mind Crystal's differentiation between prosodic abnormalities which are phonetic or phonological in origin, ataxic dysarthria would appear to fall into a phonetic category, rather than into a phonological classification. It is recognized that one function of the cerebellum is very much concerned with timing aspects of behaviour and the abnormalities described are paralleled in other movements. That is to say the prosodic features which render speech production so abnormal are the outcome of a generalized neuromuscular incoordination.

Netsell and Kent (1976) discussing a case of paroxysmal ataxic dysarthria (this is an episodic form of the condition which remits and reappears at regular and frequent intervals) suggest a monitoring function for the cerebellum. This applies to the coordinating movement of the articulatory organs. The cerebellum may issue the appropriate motor commands to achieve articulatory targets which are generated by the cerebral cortex. Kornhuber (1964) also regards the cerebellum as fulfilling a refining role.

Ataxic dysarthria presents therefore predominantly as a disorder of time, pitch and stress. The studies described have shown that misarticulation brought about by limited movement of oral musculature is also a feature, but this is generally thought to be secondary to the dysprosody. Darley, Aronson and Brown (1975) also include harsh voice quality among the clusters of deviance in this condition. Presumably this is associated with hypotonia which results in erratic and inadequate breath support for phonation.

Peripheral (Lower Motor Neurone) Dysarthria

Descriptions of the varying types of dysarthria have all related to upper motor neurone lesions. These descriptions have purposely emphasized its nature as a disorder of motor programming. Diseases of the lower motor neurone produce a wide variety of speech disorder, ranging from mild almost imperceptible dysarthria through to complete anarthria. They differ from upper motor neurone disorders however, in that they are concerned with impairment of individual movements and not with the planning and execution of movement coordinates. Canter in fact uses the terms *peripheral* and *central* as a basis for differential classification (1967, quoted by Rosenbek and La Pointe, 1978).

Lesions of the *lower motor neurone* may affect any of the components of the motor unit, the cranial nerve nuclei, nuclei in the anterior horn of the spinal cord, the motor tracts, end plates, myoneural junctions and the muscle fibres supplied by the motor unit.

Flaccidity and weakness of muscles is characteristic of this type of lesion and this may well be discrete, depending on which nuclei are involved. It is therefore possible, for example, to sustain a unilateral impairment of the hypoglossal nerve producing a unilateral paresis of the tongue. However, any resulting speech disorder is likely to be transient. It is surmounted by compensatory action of the unaffected structures so that though the configuration of movement may be unorthodox the acoustic result is acceptable. This probably entails a redesigning of motor schemata aided by external feedback through sensory channels to enable the laying down of new adaptive patterns.

Aetiology of lower motor neurone conditions is varied; it may be viral (a once common cause was *poliomyelitis*), degenerative or vascular. In the case of *myasthenia gravis* it is biochemical and is brought about by the faulty transmission of acetylcholine at the myoneural junction.

Motor neurone disease (Bulbar palsy) is a generic term for the condition which results from damage to several cranial nerve nuclei and their motor units. The speech disorder associated with these conditions is *flaccid dysarthria*. It is a secondary outcome of the primary muscle weakness and depending on which nerves are impaired, may involve the whole of the vocal tract in varying degree, so that there may be weakness of respiration, phonation, resonance and articulation.

Hypernasality is a salient feature of the disorder; dysfunction of the palatopharyngeal musculature caused by damage to the vagus (Xth) nerve is usually the cause. Incompetence of the sphincteric action may be sufficiently severe to prevent any closure between the naso and oropharynx so that there is audible nasal emission of air on phonation. Not only is resonance affected but because of the weakened egressive air stream, intraoral pressure is reduced and there is insufficient breath support for articulation. Sounds requiring a high degree of pressure, such a plosives and fricatives are particularly affected.

Additionally articulation may be affected by weakness of lips, tongue and jaws arising from involvement of the facial VII, hypoglossal XII and trigeminal V nerves. The effect is, of course, more severe if damage is bilateral. Enderby (1980) in her assessment scheme for dysarthrias carried out a number of interscorer reliability trials and a preliminary standardization on a normal adult population. This has led to modification of the initial protocol and a further standardization procedure is under way. In the meantime at the time of publication she has reported its use with over 100 dysarthric subjects. Results are recorded in bar graph form. Fig. 13 represents a profile of a typical case of bulbar palsy. The patient, a woman aged 65, sustained a cerebrovascular accident in March 1981. Initially she had some dysphasic symptoms but these were transient. The profile represents the speech status four months post onset.

The following levels are most adversely affected:

Respiration: this is shallow and irregular so that spontaneous speech is commonly in the form of short phrases and sentences. There is frequent intake of air.

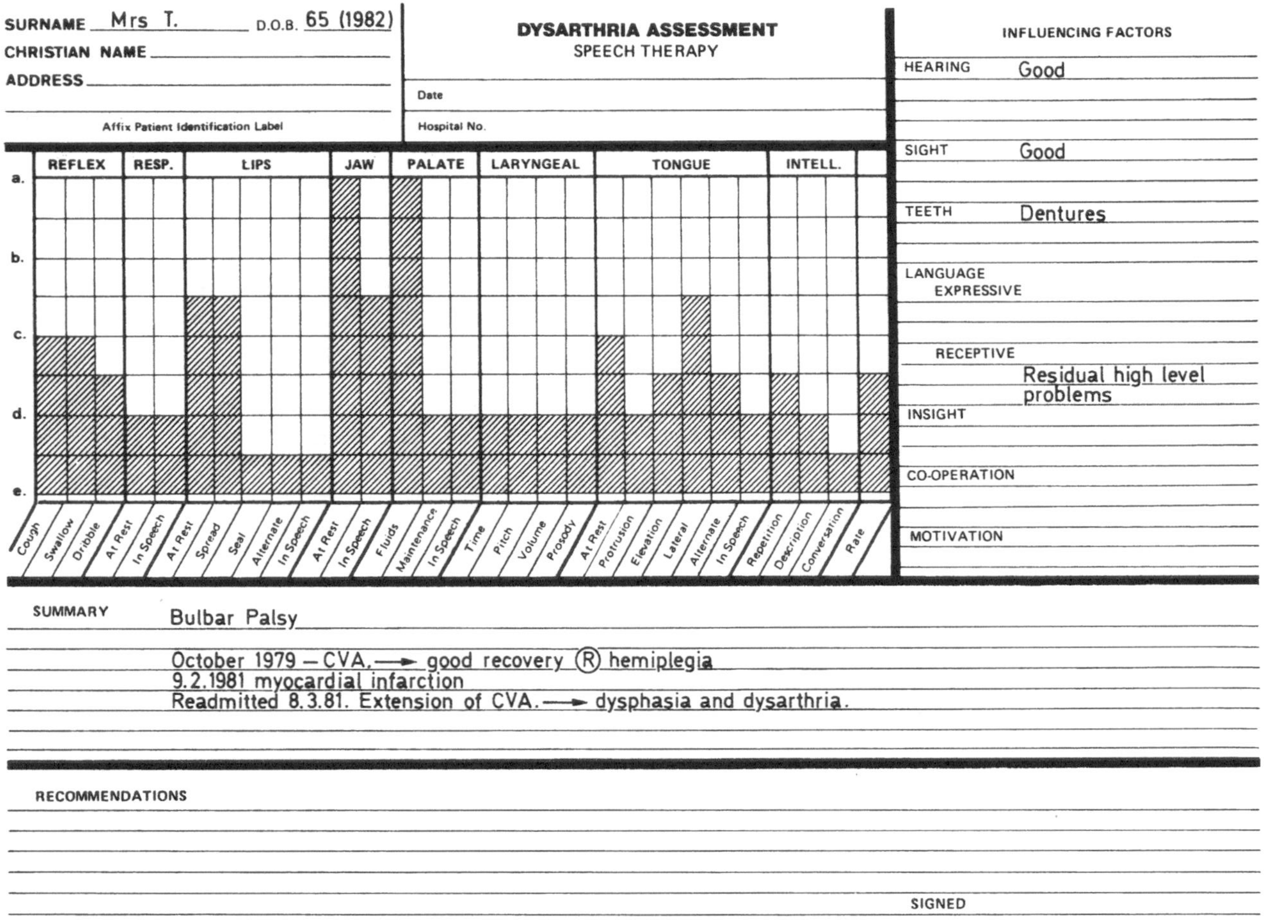

Fig. 13. Profile of patient with dysarthria associated with bulbar palsy. *a b c d e* represent increasing levels of deficit. For description of speech, refer to text. (Frenchay Dysarthria Assessment. Dr. P. Enderby)

Lip movement: at rest, lips are habitually apart and firm closure is difficult to sustain as is alternating movement when required to repeat /u,i/. Though contact can be made for bilabial plosives /p,b/ there is little acoustic effect of impounded air being released.

Palatal movement is limited and sustained raising on prolonged production of [ɑ] is impossible.

Prosodic properties of time, pitch and loudness are all abnormal.

Phonation is creaky due to aperiodic vocal fold vibration and also breathy reflecting weakness of adduction.

Tongue movement is very limited in all parameters.

While the patient can repeat very short phrases and individual words with a moderate degree of intelligibility, ongoing speech is for the most part unintelligible. Her condition is relatively static. Motivation is not very high and she does not appear to be unduly frustrated by her handicap; functional communication is adequate in a very limited sense for the quiet retiring life she leads with her husband. Speech therapy is therefore now geared to maintenance of her present condition through periodic bouts of intensive therapy acting as a booster.

Mixed Dysarthrias

Subsumed under this heading are those disorders which are the outcome of multiple lesions which generally involve both upper and lower motor neurones. The predominant features of the dysarthria will be associated with the focal site(s) of the lesions. Among the most commonly occurring types of mixed dysarthria is that resulting from *multiple sclerosis.* This is a progressive demyelinating disease affecting the white matter of the central nervous system. Aetiology is not really known; possibly it is viral in origin or it may be immunological. It causes widespread and diffuse damage throughout the central nervous system (CNS). Often it is characterized by periods of remission and exacerbation but sometimes (possibly a different type) it is straightforwardly progessive.

Speech may not be affected until later stages of the disease, though obviously this depends on the course and siting of the demyelinating process. Because of its mixed nature no one type of dysarthria emerges as a hallmark of the condition. However, it does seem that the most frequently noted features are those of ataxic dysarthria affecting nonsegmental aspects of speech.

Amyotrophic lateral sclerosis is a progressive degenerative condition with speech impairment which incorporates features of both spastic and flaccid dysarthria.

Wilson's disease is another form of mixed dysarthria. This is also a progressive degenerative condition and it arises from faulty copper metabolism. If diagnosed sufficiently early, however, the condition is reversible with appropriate diet and medication. The Mayo Clinic Study found no evidence of lower motor neurone involvement in any of the 20 patients in their series. Predominant features were spasticity, rigidity and ataxia. These were present either separately or in combinations of varying predominance.

Depending on dominance of features the dysarthria closely resembled that of pseudobulbar palsy, hypokinetic or ataxic dysarthria. Spasticity and rigidity were, however, the most marked features.

Although the foregoing descriptions of different types of dysarthria have tried to delineate characteristic symptoms, no one description can measure the totality of the communication impairment which far exceeds the sum of the separate features. Added to the description must be psychosocial factors which may adversely affect potential for recovery. Where there is widespread cerebral damage arising from trauma, for example, personality changes often constitute a barrier to the patient's recovery and the picture gained from assessment may vary considerably according to motivation and degree of cooperation. For these reasons while a thorough analysis of speech is absolutely essential, it must be seen in the context of a knowledge and understanding of the patient's pathological condition which may have had long lasting effects on health and on personality. Low thresholds of fatigue, for example, are a frequent adjunct of dysarthria and unless this is taken into account any evaluation is likely to contain spurious data which provide a false picture of capability.

Changes in Speech Production with Advancing Age

Over the past decade or so one of the most marked changes in the speech therapist's caseload has been the greatly increased number of elderly people requiring treatment. This type of patient brings problems because, as yet, knowledge about what constitutes normal change with ageing is still fragmentary. In many cases where there is no demonstrable pathology, there is nevertheless a "falling off" in cognitive skills, in memory and in many aspects of speech perception and production. Until we have precise data about this normal drift towards deterioration, standardized evaluations applicable to a younger population are unlikely to supply useful information upon which remedial programmes may be built.

Physiologically changes come about in the vocal tract through structural alterations, mainly those produced by ossification and calcification. They result in reduced efficiency in respiration and phonation whether or not there is associated respiratory disease (an additional common hazard) (Greene, 1980, 1982). Such structural changes in laryngeal cartilages may also be concomitant with alteration in mucosa of the vocal folds stemming from endocrine changes (Luchsinger and Arnold, 1965).

In supralaryngeal structures there may be skeleto-muscular change. Dental problems are common and even if not actually edentulous the elderly person may experience atrophy of alveolar tissue so that retention of dentures is difficult.

Franks (1982) writing about orofacial changes in senescence refers to a reported decrease with age in the number of myelinated fibres in the peripheral nervous system. Neuromotor function is also affected by reduced conductivity of nerves.

A number of studies, e.g. Landt (1975) have demonstrated diminution of ability to recognize form and shape intraorally in later years and also a failing skill in coordinating oral musculature for tasks requiring fine adjustment.

Israel (1973) reports two differing patterns of change in craniofacial proportions with advancing age. In the first there is a diminution in overall dimensions particularly so in the mandibular region, caused by bone resorption; conversely there may be alteration induced by progressive growth of skeletal structures.

Possibly these two conditions offer a partial explanation of differing changes in pitch direction which occur in old age. In some elderly people there is a perceptible lowering of the fundamental frequency of the voice; this could be the result of growth with a lowering of the larynx and a lengthening of the vocal tract (Laver, 1980). Other elderly people appear to have a progressively higher pitch. Shakespeare in "As You Like It" described this condition graphically as:

"the big manly voice,
turning again towards childish treble,
pipes and whistles in his sound"

and this may be associated with a shortening of the vocal tract by the raising of the larynx (through skeletal shrinkage) and atrophy of the perioral muscles. Changes in the mucosa which alter the mass of the vocal folds are also contributory.

A decreased rate of speaking has been noted along with diminished clarity of articulation. This may be due to loss of compliance in oral structures but there might well be other nonorganic reasons. The subjects of studies have in many cases been elderly people who are institutionalized. In such cases low motivation and depression could equally well be causative factors. Hearing loss must also be taken into account.

Ageing speech has been described as being at the normal end of a continuum which at its most severely impaired merges into dysarthria, notably parkinsonian hypokinetic dysarthria, Ryan and Burk (1974). Dopaminergic changes have been found to take place in many elderly people.

Alzheimer's disease formerly regarded as presenile dementia is now a term applied to a particular constellation of clinical symptoms regardless of age. It commonly presents with speech disorders though these, if specific, tend towards dyspraxic and dysphasic breakdown rather than dysarthria. Often however, the disorder is a sequel of intellectual deterioration. Alzheimer's disease too has been described as presenting the extreme of a normal process of ageing and this view is supported by autopsy evidence which shows that difference in brain tissue of the normal elderly and Alzheimer's subjects are quantitative and not qualitative.

Very little is known about the speech changes which take place with accompanying dementia. Some study has been undertaken of change in content but there are other changes in actual production of speech which as yet are undocumented. A study of these might well help towards a better understanding of the normal changes which presage the ageing process. Arie (1982) makes a strong plea for a study of such conditions.

Conclusion

Research over the last few years has brought about a radical change in attitudes of speech scientists and speech pathologists to dysarthria – this may succinctly be described as a change from the static to the dynamic. But research is still in its early stages. Speculation about neurophysiological and neurolinguistic programmes needs to be supported by clinical evidence. Detailed case studies which use discriminatively the wealth of instrumentation becoming available, to support perceptual judgement may well confirm, reject or build upon current hierarchical models.

Correlates of Verbal Dyspraxia 5

In 1861 Paul Broca described his patient "Tan" as having lost "the memory for the procedure one has to follow in order to articulate words". This condition he called *aphemia* but subsequently it became known as *Broca's aphasia*. Broca described a disorder in which the patient could understand spoken language, ideas were intact and he could recognize words and phrases which he could not pronounce nor repeat. Subsequent autopsy of Tan's brain revealed a lesion in the area of the third convolution of the frontal left lobe (later designated Broca's area). The features of this disorder parallel some of those associated with what later on became known as *dyspraxia of speech* or *verbal dyspraxia*. By annexing the word *aphasia* to Broca's name a linguistic as against motoric connotation was apparent and this sparked off a volley of controversy which has been maintained with fervour ever since.

Controversy is further compounded by the plethora of terms which denote this condition. These include *cortical dysarthria, anarthria* (Lebrun, Buyssens, and Henneaux, 1973) *phonetic disintegration, afferent motor aphasia* and *efferent motor aphasia* (Luria). For the present discussion the term *verbal dyspraxia* will be employed.

Two main sources of difference appear to keep the arguments going. They are discussed at length in Buckingham's 1979 review article. First there is the division of view as to whether the site and nature of the lesion producing dyspraxia is a localized one or whether it occurs as a result of a disconnection between language areas within the brain. Second and closely related to the first is whether the disorder is one of motor programming or whether linguistic processes are also implicated.

Darley, Aronson and Brown with their associates have, over the years, published a number of papers on dyspraxia of speech culminating in the report of the Mayo Clinic Study in 1975. In this they affirm their view of the condition as a motor disorder which does not directly involve linguistic parameters.

The strongest opposition to the motor theory probably comes from Martin (1974) who offers an alternative explanation for the disorder which he designates as an *aphasic phonological disorder*. Martin contends as indeed do many other workers that motor and linguistic processes are so closely interrelated that it is not possible to separate them in this way.

Difference of view about the type of lesion comes on the one hand from the connectionist school led by Geschwind (1965, 1975). This holds that dyspraxia is the result of a disruption *between* posterior comprehension and anterior motor zones. The centrist school, on the other, as exemplified by Luria (1970), Darley *et al.* (1975) subscribes to the view of a discrete anatomically defined lesion.

This chapter by drawing on clinical studies attempts to show that there is evidence for both a motor (phonetic) and a linguistic (phonological) interpretation of the disorder, the two aspects of dysfunction sometimes cooccurring in varying degrees and with differential patterns of recovery. But first in order to put this view into perspective it is necessary to examine in more detail some current ideas.

Motor Theory

Darley *et al.* (1975) in their model (hereinafter referred to as the Mayo model) propose three central components within the domain of language. These are the *central language processor,* the *auditory speech processor* and the *motor speech programmer.*

The central language processor receives afferent stimuli from different sensory modalities and integrates them with past experience stored in long-term memory. Its function is to transfer abstract language into meaningful linguistic form for public utterance. To achieve this it needs access to a linguistic store for the selection of appropriate units. The central language processor may correspond to the combined intentional and linguistic planning level in the neurolinguistic model described in Chapter 3. Liepmann (1900) in his delineation of different types of dyspraxia would have identified ideational dyspraxia as a breakdown at this level, that is, a condition in which the overall plan of action cannot be determined. For Darley *et al.,* however, any impairment of the central language processor is a dysphasia which they define as a unitary disorder of language (here differentiated from speech). Anatomically, they suggest that the central language processor may be in the posterior portion of the dominant temporal lobe with undetermined parts of the mid temporal, inferior parietal and anterior occipital lobes also involved. This area corresponds more or less with Liepmann's hypothesized ideational area.

The auditory speech processor appears to function as a selector of specific linguistic units which are passed to the motor speech programmer. It functions in the region of the mid temporal lobe. A lesion here would produce errors in selection of linguistic units with resulting phonemic paraphasia. The particular form of this model places the auditory speech processor *before* the central language processor in sequence of events. A "bottom up" rather than a "top down" approach is thereby suggested, this differs from many neurolinguistic theories whereby the intention and abstract linguistic programme precedes the selection of linguistic units. This model, however, in some degree circumvents the thorny problem of phonological paraphasia/dyspraxia since errors are assigned unequivocally to the language category and therefore are classified as dysphasic.

Impairment of the motor speech programmer is the only condition which the Mayo school accepts as leading to dyspraxia. They regard this component as being capable of function independent from the central language processor and therefore by implication subject to discrete damage. In relation to the neurolinguistic model described in Chapter 3 it corresponds to a combination of motor schema and neuromuscular command levels. As there is reference to a preprogramming function it seems probable that the notion of motor equivalence is accepted though it is not mentioned as such. Darley *et al.* state (1975): "The task for the trained motor speech programmer, then would be the activation of the appropriate pre-programmed chains in the appropriate order" (p. 258). Dyspraxia arising from breakdown of the motor speech programmer would correspond to Liepmann's classification of limb-kinetic apraxia and would result from a lesion of Broca's area.

The Mayo school lays considerable emphasis on articulatory disintegration as a salient feature of dyspraxia. This emphasis is somewhat puzzling since it suggests a discrete articulatory planning function whereas most models of motor control favour a more holistic view in which programmes for the entire vocal tract are planned. It is true that there may be a differential effect at different points of the tract, but if one accepts dyspraxia as a programming deficit then the viewpoint which differentiates articulation from phonation or resonance or. even respiration does not seen to be valid. The possibility of laryngeal dyspraxia is mentioned, but the claim is made that this is transient.

To some extent this is true since a number of patients do suffer a transient form of apraxic aphonia immediately post trauma. This often remits within a few days leaving other forms of persisting verbal dyspraxia. It may well be, however, that some types of phonatory disorder with at present unknown aetiology are in fact types of dyspraxia. A similar speculation might be made to account for what appears to be a growing clinical population presenting with hypernasal resonance of unknown origin. Some "cleft palate" clinics now have additional sessions devoted to patients who show no signs of anatomical abnormality to account for marked hypernasality. It is not suggested that these are all dyspraxic; other identifiable conditions will account for some, but there remain a few with intermittent nasality whose problem may well stem from deficits of programming and therefore of timing of velopharyngeal movement.

Prosodic dysfunction is regarded by the Mayo school as a secondary feature and as the outcome of compensatory strategies to combat the primary articulatory difficulty. Rosenbek and Wertz (1978) hold that the dysprosody is an intrinsic feature of the dyspraxia. This latter view appears the more plausible both on motoric and linguistic grounds.

If dyspraxia is regarded as a linguistic disorder in entirety or in part, then the prosodic disability is possibly an intrinsic part of the phonological dysfunction.

It is acknowledged that expressive language may be severely limited and that there is a preponderance of content over function words. This effect is, however, attributed to economy of effort by the Mayo workers. The sheer exertion of coping with difficult articulatory patterns, they contend, causes the speaker to limit his message to key words. An alternative explanation is that the severely limited syntactic form reflects a corresponding failure in syntactic comprehension (Berndt and Caramazza, 1980).

The Mayo description of dyspraxia of speech therefore, is of a severe articulatory disorder where output is effortful and is frequently accompanied by groping movements of the oral structures. There are errors of substitution, addition and prolongation and the degree of disintegration is in direct ratio to the length of utterance, multisyllabic words being the most vulnerable. Stress is equal and even, conferring a syllable timed character on speech. Intonation is flattened. Syntax is simplified and output may be described as telegraphic. Though there may be perceptual defects these are not regarded as being causative. Dyspraxia of speech is the outcome of a lesion of Broca's area; when this extends to the adjacent motor association area there may be an accompanying oral apraxia for nonspeech movements. There is no involvement at linguistic levels of planning and verbal comprehension is intact.

This last characteristic of the syndrome is regarded as being of considerable importance in planning treatment. It argues for an articulatory approach to remediation rather than a strategy based on language stimulation which would be appropriate for dysphasia.

Apart from this limitation of the syndrome to a purely motor (phonetic) definition the foregoing description offers an accurate description of some of the features of verbal dyspraxia. However, unanimity of description belies unanimity of underlying conditions and it is unfortunate that such a currently widely accepted view of dyspraxia does not take into account the growing number of studies which demonstrate the interrelationship of phonemic and phonetic disability in the condition. These will be discussed further below.

Duality of Dyspraxia

Luria's view of dyspraxia (1970, 1976) follows more closely that of Leipmann in that he recognizes two types: posterior, which he calls *afferent motor aphasia* and anterior – *efferent motor aphasia*. The latter closely corresponds to the Mayo definition of dyspraxia.

Afferent motor aphasia is the result of a lesion in the post-Rolandic area of the parietal lobe. This area is concerned with the integration of incoming stimuli along sensory channels (this presumably includes feedback from articulatory structures). An impairment in this synthesizing function produces a kinaesthetic dyspraxia in contrast to a more anterior lesion which is identified as a *kinetic* dyspraxia (Buckingham, 1979). Kinetic dyspraxia, Luria regards as a state of pathological inertia of coding properties. There is a marked difficulty in moving smoothly from one segment of speech to another, and therefore articulation may be grossly disordered. The patient with a kinaesthetic dyspraxia finds the main difficulty to be the appropriate selection of abstract phonemic units so that phonemic (literal) paraphasias may ensue.

The view favouring verbal dyspraxia as a *linguistic disorder* is largely based on evidence which seeks to show that the errors are phonemic rather than phonetic in nature and that therefore they represent an impairment of higher order planning and not necessarily one of neuromuscular dysfunction. This evidence is derived from extensive studies carried out notably by Lecours and his associates (1975, 1976) by Blumstein (1973) and by Martin and Rigrodsky (1974). Essentially these studies are based on phonological analysis of utterances of aphasic subjects with differing types of lesion (Broca, Wernicke and Conduction). Blumstein found qualitatively similar patterns of error in all types of aphasia. Lesser (1978) discussing Blumstein's study does, however, make the point that her transcriptions are broad phonetic and that as such they may not be sufficiently sensitive to indicate differences between Broca and Wernicke types. This fact, however, does not influence the evidence for an underlying common deficit in linguistic coding. More recently, Mackenzie (1982) has extended the Blumstein study and has reported two distinct types of disorder. Her nonfluent (Broca) group demonstrated errors consistent with accepted notions of "difficulty of production" in contrast to the fluent (Wernicke) group whose errors were more random in nature, Lecours' studies are also based on detailed analysis of phonological errors. By demonstrating that a series of rules operate in error production, that is, a consistency of pattern is observed, these workers contend that this is evidence of failure in linguistic planning.

Martin and Rigrodsky, however, make the point that both phonological and phonetic errors may be present.

Identification of differences between phonetic and phonemic errors has been the focus of subsequent work which has concentrated on the voice/voiceless contrast. This will be discussed below.

Whereas in his early work Brown differentiated between anterior and posterior type disorders, by 1975/76 he had rejected this idea in favour of a holistic view which suggests that there appears to be a *simultaneous realization out of a common deep structure into the final perceptual and motoric forms of the language act (JWB)*.

Such a view is in accord with that expressed in current neurophysiological theory which regards speech production as the outcome of neurological systems working coordinatively rather than sequentially and to some extent independently. It also allows for, the development of the idea that the deficit in verbal dyspraxia is not necessarily qualitatively different in relation to the site of the lesion. Blumstein's 1973 analysis demonstrated this.

It therefore seems that dyspraxia shows certain features which are "dysphasic" in nature. In some respects it also closely resembles some types of dysarthria, particularly in certain nonsegmental aspects of timing and intonation.

As Buckingham (1979) indicates, the position with regard to identification of dyspraxia is a somewhat anomalous one, in that there is this interface between the linguistic and motoric levels of speech. To quote: "We are then left in the strange position of saying that this patient population has 'an apraxia of speech' without being able to say that any one of their actual speech errors is (in itself) diagnostic of that group" (p. 222).

Plainly we are once more up against the perennial dilemma of "How shall a thing be called?"

Experienced workers, e.g. Johns and La Pointe (1976), Trost and Canter (1974) have recognized a clinical entity which in its constellation of features is different from both dysarthria and Wernicke's aphasia.

Much research has concentrated on the acquired condition but *developmental verbal dyspraxia* is also recognized by some workers as representing a particular type of disability which it is possible to differentiate from other developmental language disorders. As with the acquired condition, this view is also in dispute, and a critical review by Guyette and Diedrich (1982) suggests that at present there is insufficient evidence to substantiate the claim that it constitutes a discrete disorder. These authors consider that the assorted signs and symptoms attributed as evidence of a developmental dyspraxia can also be applied equally to other types of communicative disability in children.

There is, one must concede, a paucity of empirical data. Most of the findings are based on clinical impressions, observations and anecdotal evidence, but these should not be discounted. Rather what is needed is a much greater degree of systematic investigation; some really penetrating in-depth case studies might lend support either for or against the idea as well as doing much to overcome the speculative nature of many present views. Whether or not there is sufficient evidence to regard verbal dyspraxia as an entity, repeated reference to certain constellations of cooccurring features makes it difficult to refute utterly its existence.

Criteria for establishing a diagnosis in the developmental state are obviously very different from those in the acquired condition. In the latter there is in most cases an established pathology which is assumed to be causal. With children, developmental history is often heterogenous and inconclusive. While there may be reference in pre- and perinatal history to anomalous conditions such as anoxia, foetal distress, postmaturity etc.: these conditions also occur in the histories of children with other types of communicative disorder and indeed in those with little evidence of any sort of disorder. One must therefore be cautious in the too ready assumption of a causal link. The biological history of 13 children with features of verbal dyspraxia in an unpublished pilot study (Edwards, 1982) yielded inconclusive evidence. Only in one case was there a report of an abnormal pregnancy. This exception listed a history of urinary infection and of hemorrhage, the child subsequently being born at 42 weeks with deformities of hands and feet (a familial condition). Neurological and biochemical histories of the 13 children were varied and in no case provided a confirmatory diagnosis though there were implications of abnormalities. Two of the children had reduced muscle tone, one was reported to have had a prolonged fit at 14 months and another had febrile convulsions at 12 months and at 4 years. There was a history of language disability in other members of the family in 4 cases. One family, not part of this study, has revealed dyspraxic type disorders in 3 out of the 4 siblings and a history of speech disability in at least 5 maternal relatives (uncles, aunts and cousins).

Some of the misunderstandings and controversies in the way of accepting the notion of a "Mixed entity" may have stemmed from a Procrustean desire to fit the facts into an "either/or" classification; either motor *or* linguistic but not motor *and* linguistic. An adoption of Brown's (1975) thesis of *levels* rather than *centres* of processing may be more satisfactory.

A further difficulty of definition occurs in acquired dyspraxia in that it is frequently the result of widespread damage which also produces a dysphasia. In such cases it is not always easy to differentiate between a dyspraxic induced struggle to produce a word and a similar effect stemming from word retrieval difficulty. Again whereas most dyspraxics are nonfluent one occasionally encounters a case of superfluency where timing seems to be out control (cp. some types of dysarthria) and perseveration and contamination of adjoining segments of speech are observed. Such cases closely resemble the classic description of cluttering and also may in some respects be reminiscent of jargon dysphasia.

Some Features of Dyspraxia

Volition. A feature which is repeatedly referred to in the literature is the volitional nature of dyspraxia. Hughlings Jackson regarded this as one of the distinguishing signs of the condition, not just in relation to speech but to other movement as well. The writer recalls an adult patient who when invited to sit down, remained rooted to the spot, quite unable to initiate the sequence of necessary movements. And yet on other occasions he would come in and sit down quite naturally.

The difference between voluntary and involuntary aspects is also illustrated quite graphically by the islands of completely normal speech which are interspersed among the dyspraxic errors. Another severely dyspraxic patient with no residual dysphasic signs, in the midst of a struggle to express some point, when asked where he had parked his car, replied with absolute clarity: *"I didn't bring it today, I've sold it. I came b-b-by b-b-bus"*, before lapsing again into dyspraxic struggle.

Variability of response is another feature, often noted in relation to speech. This variability is reported to be one of the features differentiating dysarthria from dyspraxia. Within the bounds of mood and fatigue the dysarthric person will produce similar responses on consecutive occasions. Not so the dyspraxic. The Mayo patient's successive attempts at the word *tornado* provides a classic example. The audiorecording demonstrates about 12 attempts at the word each effort differing from the others yet all broadly conforming to the sounds within the word. Children too show similar inconsistencies. Following, is a transcript of an eight-year old's attempt to come to grips with *arithmetic:*

Therapist: "Let's try arithmetic"		[ʌ'rɪθmʌtɪk]
A		[ʌ'mɛɪ'tɪ'kɪk]
T	repeats	
A		[ʌ'ʊɪθ'mɪ'kɪt]
T	together walking one	[ʌrɪθmʌtɪk]
A	step/syllable	[ʌʊɪθmʌtɪk]
A		
A	say it again	[ʌʊɪʔmʌtɪk]
A		[ʌ'wʌ'tɪ'mɪk]
A		[ʌ'wʌ'wɪ'tɪmɪk]
A		[ʌ'ʊ'ɪθɪmɪt].

It will be observed that progressive repetition does not bring approximation to the target. Modelling and the provision of a strong beat help but without these the child loses the syllabic integrity of the word.

Examples of variability produced by other children are:

umbrella	→	[ʌrʌbelʌ, bʌrʌmeʌ, ʌmbelʌ]	7 year-old boy
particular	→	[kɪ, kutɪkɪu, kukɪkɪku]	8 year-old boy
canary	→	[kɪnmɛəri, kənɛəri, kɪnɪkɪ]	6 year-old boy

Here too there is inappropriate stress. But the errors are not random and the realization can be related to the target or to some other sound within the word. In acquired conditions there is also evidence of systematic rules being employed in error production.

Developmental verbal dyspraxia is frequently though not invariably associated with *clumsiness*. Early studies in the 1960s in fact focussed on these aspects with only a passing reference to the speech disorder (Walton, Ellis and Court, 1962; Dare and Gordon, 1970). Edwards found that among the 13 children in her pilot study 10 revealed clumsiness of gross and/or fine motor movements.

There may also be an accompanying oral motor dyspraxia but it must be emphasized that the two conditions, i.e. verbal and oral dyspraxia can be and often are quite discrete. There is therefore no way in which the cause of the verbal deficit can be attributed to the impairment in oral movement.

Learning difficulties may also be reported though it is not clear whether there is a causal relationship between these and verbal dyspraxia. In fact, the cooccurrence of this constellation of symptoms has led to the adoption of the term "Clumsy Child Syndrome" (Gubbay, 1975; Gordon and McKinley, 1980).

The plasticity of the developing brain is another factor which makes the establishment of a firm neurological diagnosis difficult. Guyette and Diedrich (1981) state that a confirmed diagnosis would only be possible if there were bilateral damage. They base this statement on the assumed capacity for compensation of the other nondominant hemisphere. However, this assumed compensatory ability may have been over estimated in a number of studies because of insufficiently sensitive language assessment. Woods and Carey (1978) found signs of residual linguistic impairment in children who had sustained nonprogressive left cerebral lesions. This appeared when the trauma had occurred as early as 4 years 7 months of age.

One of the principal factors to be considered is the different language status of the child who is acquiring language and the adult who has suffered a dissolution of a previously intact language system.

However, despite lack of correspondence in many aspects of the conditions, developmental verbal dyspraxia and acquired verbal dyspraxia do share certain common features.

Linguistic Features of Dyspraxia

Dyspraxic errors in their features of inconsistency and misordering bear a considerable resemblance to the phonemic paraphasias of dysphasic patients. In neurolinguistic terms this might be explained as a failure of coordination between the motor schema and neuromuscular command levels of planning. Laver (1977) notes this stage as being a likely source of error in slips of the tongue. From the admittedly limited corpus of dyspraxic errors currently available there are grounds for comparing these with slips of the tongue phenomena. Samples obtained from the 13 children in the developmental study do not include any phonotactically unacceptable realizations. For the most part, they are within-word errors rather than within-tone group because most of the children were nonfluent. Boomer's and Laver's (1968) examples were of errors which occurred within or across tone groups and Laver suggests that they may arise from asynchrony between the components of the planning system. The initial stages of the linguistic program planned in sequences of tone groups is relatively faster than the later articulatory stage. A sort or "stacking up" of tone groups might well lead to sequential errors.

One of the comparatively rare examples of a superfluent dyspraxic child did show an across-group errors:

"the teacher I'm with is drawing / ... these kind of circles / and some different kind of *clocks* / and her *cl-paw – drawed pointers* / while I tell the time."

This illustrates very well a perseverative "cl" error and an anticipatory "paw" error.

An alternative explanation is that this type of error originates in the very early stages of the linguistic programme, in fact, in the selection of the linguistic units.

La Pointe, Horner and Johns (1975) analysed phonemic errors made by a group of dyspraxic adults. They found examples of *anticipatory, perseverative* and *metathetic,* i.e. transposition of sounds, realizations.

The developmental study also included examples of this type of error:

vegetables	→	[edʒbʌtlz]	(anticipatory)
ambulance	→	[æmbi'lbʌns]	(perseverative)
buttercup	→	'[kʌtəbʌp]	(metathetic)

One of the features characterizing dyspraxia most frequently cited is that of inconsistency. This is, however, a qualified term in that it applies only to specific word errors. That is to say that during connected speech, whether reading or spontaneous the same words will tend to present difficulty though the actual errors made will vary. All 13 children in the developmental study showed this type of variability.

There is some evidence of linguistic rules operating in dyspraxic utterances. Such evidence favours its interpretation as a disorder of linguistic programming without necessarily ruling out the possibility of motor programming deficits existing as well.

Blumstein (1973), basing her evidence on data from 17 aphasic patients, noted a preponderance of errors involving one distinctive feature only. Among these she observed a hierarchy of difficulty. Errors of voicing were frequent, particularly in the direction of voiced to voiceless. Cluster reduction and addition of sounds were also noted.

Trost and Canter (1974) have also undertaken major studies of Broca dysphasics. They report a similar pattern of error and Trost also emphasizes the evidence of underlying linguistic planning.

Samples from Edwards' developmental study also support these findings:

biscuits   →   [gɪsgɪts]

change of one feature in word initial position
voicing of second element of cluster

fork   →   [kɔ, fkɔt]

deletion of final consonant which now appears in word initial position
insertion of additional consonant which should appear in word final position

word final consonant changed in one feature
bath   →   [bæs̬]
addition of one feature (stridency) in word final position.

Hardcastle and Morgan (1982) used electropalatography (EPG) and pneumotachography is investigate tongue dynamics and voice onset time in a number of children with articulatory/phonological disorders. One of their subjects, a 13 year-old boy was diagnosed as dyspraxic with a moderate degree of dysarthria some hearing loss and mild mental handicap (the criteria for diagnosis are not described).

His main difficulty was reported to be a failure in coordinating oral movements both for speech and nonspeech activities.

The EPG reading revealed him to be producing alveolar and palato-alveolar consonants as velar sounds /t → k, d → g, h → k/. However, as well as posterior contact between velum and the back of the tongue there was also normal alveolar – tongue tip contact, though this was not recognized perceptually. Fig. 14 shows the printout of tongue movement for the word *tent*. Each frame represents the output from 64 electrodes, with the small squares indicating areas of tongue contact. The velar area is at the top of the frame and alveolar at the bottom. Sampling is at 10 ms intervals.

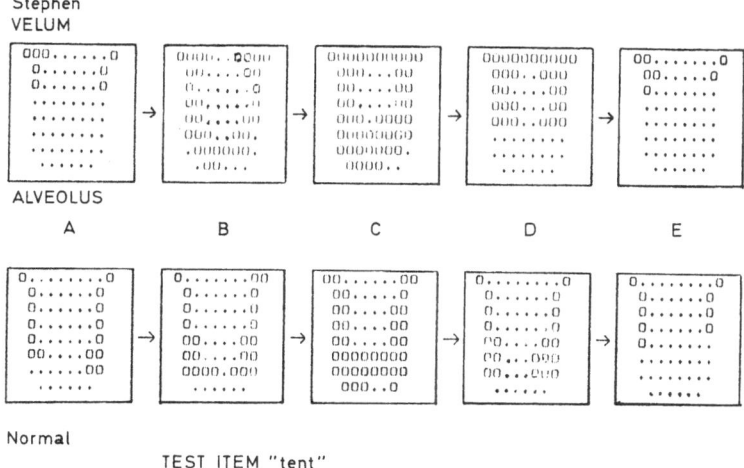

Fig. 14. Electropalatography showing abnormal and normal articulation. Each diagram represents one frame of the computer printout and shows the position of the 64 electrodes. The printout is read from left to right and is taken at 10 ms intervals. The rectangles show the tongue contacts made during the production of the alveolar obstruent [t] in initial position. (Reproduced by permission of Dr. W. J. Hardcastle, R. A. Morgan and British Journal of Disorders of Communication)

One of the other deviant features in this particular subject was in *voicing* and this is one of the most frequently cited errors in dyspraxic disorders. It has been the subject of many investigations to establish differentiation between phonemic and phonetically determined error. The voice onset time for Hardcastle's and Morgan's subject is illustrated in Fig. 15a. Comparison with normal readings (Fig. 15b) over six productions of plosives t,d; p,b; and k,g; shows marked overlap for p,b and in k,g, there is little difference in the voice onset time.

Voicing onset time anomalies have been described in other dyspraxia studies. Yoss and Darley (1974) found a high incidence of this error in the group they tentatively labeled as having developmental apraxia of speech; it occurred with twice the frequency which might be expected in children with delayed language development. Williams, Ingham and Rosenthal (1981),

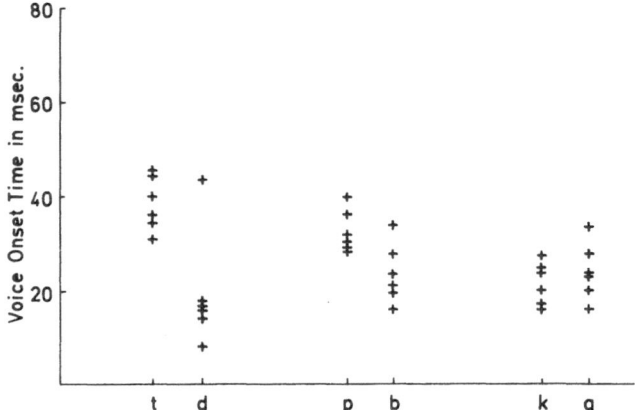

Fig. 15a. Graph showing distribution in a dyspraxic child's VOT values for six repetitions of each of the plosives t, d, p, b, k, g

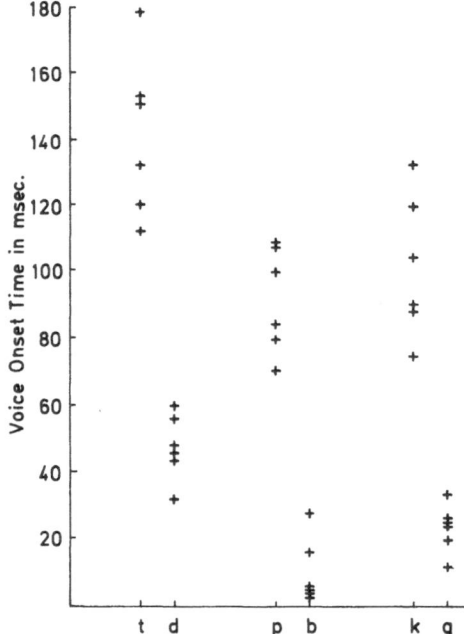

Fig. 15b. Graph showing distribution of normal subject's VOT values (in ms) for six repetitions of each of the plosives t, d, p, b, k, g. (Reproduced by permission of Dr. W. J. Hardcastle, R. A. Morgan and British Journal of Disorders of Communication)

however, in a replication of the Yoss and Darley study failed to confirm this finding. Edwards noted voicing errors in 8 out of 13 children in her developmental study. Examples are:

ball   →   [pɔl]
duck   →   [tʊk]
two   →   [du]
paper   →   [beɪdə]

Freeman, Sands and Harris (1978) studied VOT in a dyspraxic subject whose speech included voicing feature errors. They compared spectrographic data of normal production of voiceless stop consonants with their voiced cognates. As with Hardcastle's and Morgan's subject, there was a failure to observe the discrete temporal difference between voiced and voiceless sounds. Spectrographic readings confirmed perceptual judgements which indicated that about 50% of /p/ productions were perceived as /b/, 35% of /k/ as g and 25% of /g/ as /k/. Freeman *et al.* compare these findings with developmental data and interpret them as supporting Jakobson's regression hypothesis (1968).

In 1980, Blumstein, Cooper, Goodglass, Statlender and Gottlieb published the results of an experimental study in which they examined VOT values in 18 subjects. 13 were aphasic (4 Broca, 4 Conduction and 5 Wernicke) 1 was dysarthric and 4 were normal controls. The dysarthric patient had a traumatic brain stem encephalopathy.

One of the principal aims of the study was to examine the incidence and pattern of phonetic and phonemic errors. A phonemic error they defined as one in which the VOT value of the target fell within the VOT range of the opposite category. A phonetic error would occur when the VT values fell between and/or outside the normal value for the voiced *and* voiceless categories.

Results indicated that the Broca group made the highest percentage of errors, most of these being phonetic, Wernicke subjects made few errors and these were equally phonetic and phonemic Conduction subjects made slightly more phonetic than phonemic errors. The phonetic errors when compared with those made by the dysarthric patient show differences. VOT for voiceless sounds in the dysarthric is considerably longer and there is no overlap between voiced and voiceless production. These data lend support to the view that in contrast to dysarthria the phonetic errors made by the Broca (dyspraxic) patients do not reflect low level neuromuscular impairment but rather a higher order articulatory planning disorder and that many are akin to aphasic errors. These could be at the abstract motor schema level described in Chapter 3.

Itoh and his colleagues (1982) on the other hand in a series of studies, as a result of comparison between apraxic, fluent aphasic and normal subjects on a measure of VOT concluded that differences were due to disturbed control over timing of laryngeal and supralaryngeal movement. They did not find the similarities in the different types of aphasia reported by Blumstein and her associates.

7*

Stress and Timing

Prosody is reported to be abnormal in most of the studies. As already stated, Darley *et al.* (1975) regard this as secondary to the primary articulatory disorder while Rosenbek (1978) includes "prosodic disturbance among the primary symptoms" (p. 199). Blumstein noted dysprosody as one of the differentiating features between her sample of Broca patients (which included dyspraxics) and the Wernicke asphasics with phonological impairment, though she did not specify the nature of the difference. Mackenzie did not investigate prosody in her study.

A conclusion about the source of the prosodic disturbance in dyspraxia is problematical, that is, whether it is a *prosodic disability* and *linguistic,* or a *dysprosody* and *motoric* (Crystal's 1981 terminology). The third possibility that it comprises elements of both aspects is the most plausible and one which accords with the emerging picture of dyspraxia as a type of "halfway house" disorder in which elements of dysarthria and dysphasia may cooccur.

Only one of the 13 children in the pilot study (Edwards) was able to signal changes in stress and rhythm appropriately. This failure, potentially has a far reaching effect on language, since a stress timed language like English relies on contrastive stress to signal changes in meaning. The children were required to imitate a model where a change in stress altered meaning:

The tractor crashed into the red car.
The tractor crashed into the *red* car.
The tractor crashed into the red *car.*
The *tractor* crashed into the red car.
The tractor *crashed* into the red car.

Imitations were generally syllable timed with equal and even stress on all words.

Neither were the children able to signal appropriate intonation contrasts. Imitation of

a cup of còffee please,
can you càtch the báll?

resulted in no variation between statement and question.

Spontaneous speech which was sparse, showed abnormal pause and prolongation of vowels, so that overall timing rules were not observed. The superfluent dyspraxics seemed to be unable to "turn take" in normal conversational interchange. They always tended to start before the other speaker had finished and in rote tasks where a finite sample was requested, as for example in counting 1–10 they would continue 11, 12, 13 and so on. Similarly with reciting days of the week they would start again with *Sunday* after completing the cycle.

Itoh, Sasanuma and Ushijima (1979) and Itoh *et al.* (1980) used fibreoptics and an X-ray microbeam system with pellet tracking techniques in two experiments in which they were able to evaluate simultaneously velar, lip and tongue movements of a patient with acquired dyspraxia of speech. Results showed temporal asynchrony between the articulators in ongoing speech. Three repetitions of the Japanese word *deenee* in a carrier phrase showed a different time relationship between velar and tongue tip movement each time. In the first, tongue tip rise and velar lowering for /n/ were synchronous; in the second, the velum was lowered *prior* to the elevation of the tip and in the third the velum made a minimal descent so that the /n/ was perceptually denasalized.

Velocity of lip movement in rapid repetition of *pa pa pa* was considerably slower than that of a normal control. It also differed from normal slow repetition whose chief characteristic is a prolonged closure period.

Itoh *et al.* (1980) compared their readings with similar data obtained from a subject with ataxic dysarthria and also one with amyotrophic lateral sclerosis. As might be predicted these readings also showed marked abnormalities. In this particular publication only velocity of lip movement is reported for the dysarthrics; other readings are described in Hirose *et al.* (1977, 1978) (in Japanese). There were marked differences between the control and other subjects and this related particularly to regularity of closure, the ataxic dysarthric showing extreme irregularity.

In the earlier study Itoh and his colleagues observed velar movements during speech of the same dyspraxic subject by means or a fibrescopic system. A detailed phonological investigation of the patient's speech had previously been carried out 7 months post onset of a cerebro vascular accident (CVA) lesion affecting the tip of the sylvian fissure and subjacent white matter in the left (dominant) temporal lobe. This first investigation took place in 1971. Findings had at that time not shown aphasia but a marked phonological disorder characterized predominantly by errors of anticipation, perseveration and metathesis. This led one of the workers, Sasanuma, to suggest that "the impairment might not be confined to the motor aspects of speech, but might be extended into the linguistic (but almost exclusively phonological) spheres as well" (p. 229).

Six years later the fibrescopic investigation took place. There now remained only residual overt traces of the previous dyspraxia. Findings indicated considerable variability in timing of velar movement on successive repetition of words when compared with a normally speaking control. Sequential movements of the velum were, however, well preserved. There was also evidence of movement associated with coarticulation indicating operation of a feedforward scanning mechanism. These authors interpret the findings as being indicative of a motor planning disorder in which synchronized movement of the articulators is disturbed. Taking the long-term history and evaluations, the implication is that the patient presented originally with a predominantly phonological disorder, but over the course of time this had resolved leaving a residual phonetic disorder. Although there are obvious limitations in single case studies of this type, the findings are nevertheless of considerable interest in that they favour a view of dyspraxia as a mixed disorder.

Rhythmicity

Impaired rhythmicity has been reported in a number of child studies in relation to language disability (Kracke, 1975; Lee, 1980). Tasks have usually been based on recognition and replication of rhythmic patterns. In a graded test in which children were required to imitate successively more complicated clapping patterns, Edwards found that the dyspraxic children were unable to reproduce stress and timing differences though they could often estimate correctly the total number of claps in the sequence. The arhythmicity of their nonspeech activities reflects corresponding difficulties in signalling appropriate contrasts in speech. There is apparent a lack of ability to reproduce appropriate tone groups.

The sentence:

The car/with red stripes/crashed into the tractor/

one dyspraxic boy of 13 reproduced as:

The car with red stripes/it crashed into the tractor/

Martin (1972) describes a hierarchy of rhythmic organization in which he lays emphasis on the fact that rhythm is not necessarily regular and repetitive, i.e. concatenative, but is more often relative, so that sequences of sound bear an intrinsic relationship to each other and an extrinsic one to the utterance as a whole. This view of course endorses Lenneberg's notion of the rhythmic "pacemaker".

When dyspraxia is extended to other movements a similar lack of harmonious coordination is apparent, so that in activities like hopping, kicking and throwing, threading etc. arms and legs, head and body seem to move independently.

In nonspeech oral movements also there is difficulty both in imitating and in carrying out to command, consecutive movements. This is an interesting facet because the two activities employ different sensory channels, visual and auditory, respectively. Rapid alternating tongue movement, diadochokinesis, as in repetition of the sequence /p t k/ is often impossible to achieve. Both the Yoss and Darley (1974) and the Williams *et al.* (1981) studies presented consistent results on this task and it was one of the features which Yoss and Darley felt to be important in differentiating their dyspraxic group from those with functional articulatory disorders.

Sensory Feedback

The predominance of velar sounds observed in Stephen (Hardcastle and Morgan, op.cit.) is an interesting one which has been observed clinically in other studies (Edwards, 1973; Macaluso Haynes, 1978). Although Stephen did appear to be using the tongue tip, more frequently there often appears to be a neglect of this, and this factor has been related to impaired *kinaesthetic feedback* influencing sound production in the learning stages of speech.

It has also been noted that some dyspraxics perform poorly on tasks which attempt to evaluate kinaesthetic feedback, Rosenbek, Wertz and Darley (1973) found that 18 out of a group of 30 subjects had difficulty in carrying out three tasks designed to measure orosensory perception. The remaining 12 performed adequately. They observed a direct relationship between the severity of the dyspraxia and the level of performance. The two groups might correspond with Luria's classification of two types of dyspraxia. The afferent motor type in which there is an impairment in the synthesis of incoming sensory information could equate with the 18 subjects who could not carry out the tactile kinaesthetic tasks while the efferent motor classification could apply to the 12 who experienced no difficulty.

It is rather difficult to know what degree of importance should be assigned to studies of this type. The constraints upon obtaining a true evaluation of kinaesthetic feedback have already been outlined in Chapter 3 as has the relative significance of external and internal feedback. If one accepts that both systems have a contribution to make in the programming of speech then it is possible that deviant or disrupted feedback could affect planning.

Auditory Perception

As far as can be ascertained, assessment of auditory perception has been on a fairly superficial level and in the Mayo studies, subjects were reported to score well on tests of discrimination and sequencing. But it must be stated that present methods of evaluating auditory perception of speech are not very satisfactory and this comment applies to most types of language disability. It is doubtful that naive assessments of feature discrimination come anywhere near to measuring the complexities inherent in the auditory *recognition* of spoken language. In fact, when we use present methods of assessment it is questionable whether we really know what it is we are attempting to measure. It is likely, for example, that differential processes operate for the analysis of different linguistic levels of input, phonological, syntactic and semantic. Johns' and Darley's dyspraxic subjects were able to discriminate meaningful word lists better than nonsense syllables whereas the normal controls performed equally well on both tasks. Martin (1974) suggests that this reflects "the interaction of phonological processes in the language system" (p. 59).

Verbal Comprehension

The uncertainty about the status of auditory perception in dyspraxic subjects leads also to a questioning of the assumption made throughout the earlier literature that verbal comprehension is unaffected. Perhaps it would be more accurate to say that subjects have usually performed reasonably well on *the measures of comprehension which have been presented to them*. These have traditionally been based on assessment of cognitive and not on linguistic components of comprehension. In the developmental study (Edwards, 1982) all 13 children were reported to have achieved normal or near normal scores on the comprehension scale of the Reynell Developmental Scales (RDLS experimental edition, 1969). This test reflects very much a level of conceptual understanding and does not tap syntactic levels to any great extent. In an overview of comprehension deficits in Broca's aphasia (and here the term includes dyspraxia), Berndt and Caramazza (1980) concluded that when syntactic levels were assessed differentially as in tasks requiring the understanding of ambiguous sentences, where a change in a syntactic element alters the meaning, the Broca subjects performed less well than normals. It was also suggested that there might be a direct association between this deficit and the limited syntactic output. In other words the notion of telegraphic-like speech as an economy of effort strategy is questioned.

Lesser (1978, pp. 170–176) reviews and discusses fully the relationship between comprehension and speech production.

Writing and Drawing

There may be an impairment in writing in that it demonstrates sequential reversal and spatial anomalies. However, the possibility of a perceptual deficit whereby recognition of the relationship between components of the pattern is impaired must also be considered. Laver (1977) suggests a common control function for the linguistic elements of both reading and writing, presumably at the abstract level of planning. It is only in the later neuromuscular conversion stage that there is specific differentiation. By then the errors may well be written into the program. It may be that there are linguistic and motor errors apparent in writing which parallel those which occur in speech.

These two samples of writing by dyspraxic children, while both are very defective can be seen to illustrate this idea. That produced by a girl, Fig. 16 a, shows strange reversals and sequential errors but she has some spatial sense about the way in which words occupy space on a page. The boy (Fig. 16 b), on the other hand, having copied this piece of writing and having attempted to space it out with vertical bars, still cannot succeed. The writing is crowded over on the left hand side of the page and there is really no difference in spacing between words and between letters.

Summary

So even after a detailed description of dyspraxia we are still left with a feeling of uncertainty about the nature of the condition, and the controversy surrounding it is likely to remain as active as ever. A partial resolution seems to be offered by Brown's most recent model which rejects the notion of centres for speech and the accompanying dichotomies of reception and expression, lingustic and motor, but which instead puts forward a theory of levels. In this way it is possible to see language disability as a continuum and one is spared the need to classify as *either* linguistic *or* motor. The progress of Sasanuma's

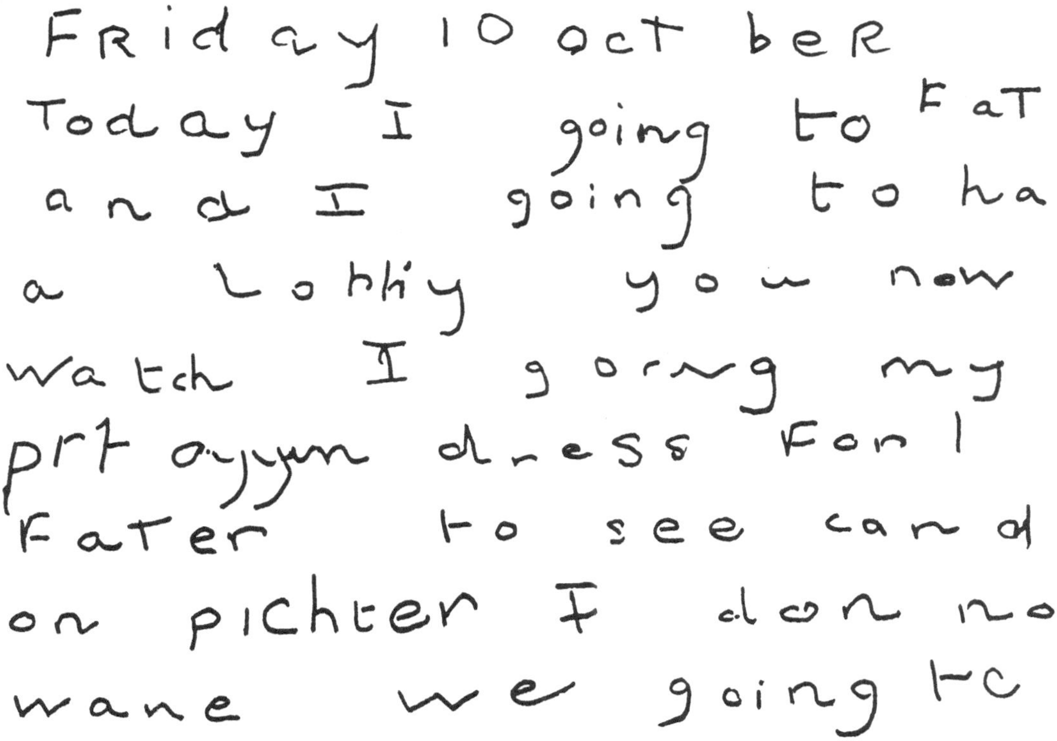

FRiday 10 octbeR
Today I going to FaT
and I going to ha
a Lohiy you now
watch I gorng my
prt ayyun dress For l
Fater to see can d
on pichter I don no
wane we going to

Fig. 16a. Today I'm going to (the theatre) and I'(m) going to ha(ve) a lolly you now watch. I'(m) going to wear my party dress for (the) theatre to see (cand?) on (the) picture I don't know when we (are) going to . . .

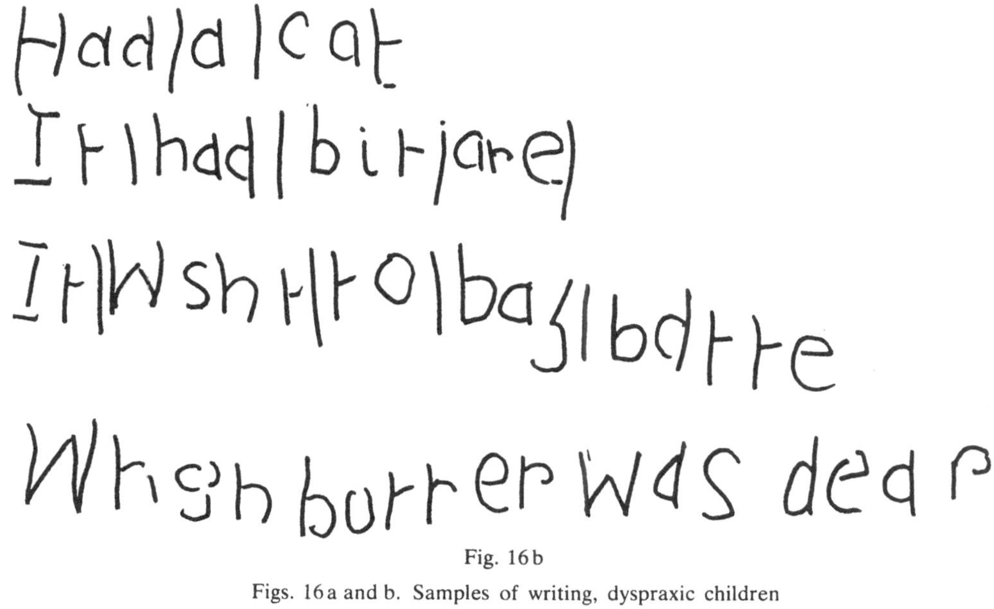

Had/a/cat
It/had/bit/are/
It/Wsh/t/o/ba/bdtte
Whsh butter Was dead

Fig. 16b

Figs. 16a and b. Samples of writing, dyspraxic children

patient from 1971 when he was first seen with a disability which at the time seemed to embody deficits of selection and retrieval through to the examination six years later when residual errors seemed representative of a more downstream level in production may serve as an example of the continuum theory.

Buckingham (1979) provides some ideas about differences which might be relevant to distinguish what he terms anterior Broca's aphasics, posterior Wernicke's aphasics and cortical dysarthrics. He cites features which are common to two or more of the conditions and on these grounds sees little merit in continuance of the term apraxia of speech. But the rejection of a term does not help very much clinically. It is recognized that a label in itself serves as little more than a convenient shorthand method of communicating essential features of a condition, provided of course that the sender and receiver understand a similar meaning by the label. In the case of *dyspraxia* this may very well not be the case.

Nevertheless speech therapists are called upon to assess and to treat patients who present with a constellation of disabilities some of which are akin to aphasic phonological disorder and some which resemble types of dysarthria, while there may also be other features which cannot confidently be placed in one or other category but seem to have affiliations with both.

Furthermore, within the domain of neuropathologically orientated disorders speech therapists stand in close professional relationship to neurologists who on the whole abide by traditionally accepted classification and terminology. Whatever detailed linguistic description may be deemed necessary and appropriate between colleagues of the same profession, there

Table 1. *Motor and linguistic errors associated with verbal dyspraxia*

Phonetic Errors	Phonological Errors
Equal and even stress	Absence or paucity of tone units and nuclear stress
Incoordinated movement of oral structures, e.g. velum → hypernasality.	Disorder of selection and retrieval of linguistic units, syntactic and phonological, e.g. nasal/nonnasal contrasts.
Phonetic errors related to hierarchy of "difficulty".	Phonological errors not related to difficulty – random.
Consistency of error.	Variability of error though tendency for different errors to occur on same words.
VOT abnormalities due to timing errors at neuromuscular level.	VOT abnormalities due to programming deficits at motor schema level.
Syllable deletion.	Syllable addition and deletion.
Vowel prolongation. Effortful sequential flow between phones.	
Associated problems of clumsiness and nonverbal dyspraxia.	

still remains a need to communicate lucidly with others. For this reason, it is unlikely that terminology of this type will fall into disuetude.

Table 1 attempts to summarize those features of verbal dyspraxia which can be considered to fall into phonetic and phonological categories. In some cases realizations can be the outcome of impairment at either level and indeed at different times in the course of recovery may represent transition from one level to another, that is to say, an initially higher order difficulty involving selection and retrieval of the linguistic programme may give way to residual difficulties at a level of articulatory programming. VOT as has been shown may be phonetic or phonological.

The differences between equal and even stress (phonetic) and absence or paucity of tone units and nuclear stress (phonological) is language specific. In a bilingual patient if the disorder is phonetic it will be apparent and replicated in other languages; if it is phonological it may be confined to one language or extending to more than one, will not necessarily manifest identical abnormalities.

More important than a preoccupation with terminology is the need for painstaking investigation of all parameters of speech so that we may build up a more comprehensive picture of the disorder. Such investigations might then resolve some of the terminological arguments as well as providing data on which to base more effective plans of therapy.

Management 6

Confronted with a radical change in ability to communicate, whether this be insidious or sudden in onset, the victim will be required to have recourse to many adaptive measures in order to survive socially. The child who has to contend with a similar level of handicap as an integral part of his development also, in a different way has to come to terms with the fact that his life in many respects will be very different from that led by the vast majority of children.

Help towards an understanding and acceptance of the disability may come in the first instance from the medical adviser, general practitioner, neurologist, paediatrician or geriatrician. But at best such support will be limited by time and likely to be offered during periodic professional visits. On a day to day basis it may well be that considerable support will be given by a member of the remedial professions whose frequent contact through treatment nourishes a close relationship with both patient and relatives.

The speech therapist is in a particularly favoured position by the very nature of the work. Application of learned techniques to functional language must come about in a conversational setting and thus must relate closely to the patient's needs and interests. Such a relationship, however, carries responsibilities and problems often not readily soluble. In particular the patient may seek an honest appraisal about the extent of disability and the likelihood of recovery.

Byers Brown's (1981) account of her patient, Mrs Black, is a poignant illustration of this situation. This patient was suffering from a progressive bulbar palsy, but until he was in a better position to predict her reaction, the consultant neurologist was not ready to discuss prognosis with the patient. While this decision had little effect on immediate short-term therapy, inevitably as time went by and a close relationship developed between clinician and patient, the question of progress or lack of it was raised. Most therapists are faced with the dilemma posed by Byers Brown. A dishonest answer would undermine future mutual confidence when the truth became apparent, while on the other hand a revelation about the likely course of the disease would be in contravention of the consultant's decision made in the interest of the patient. In the event the patient herself sought a further meeting during which all the implications of her condition were considered. This cleared the way for the therapist to teach, in an atmosphere of mutual trust and confidence, the techniques which would help the patient when the time came that her speech was no longer intelligible.

Realistic acceptance of goals is also essential for the clinician and not just for the patient. This point is strongly put by Rosenbek and La Pointe (1978) when they state that a return to complete normal speech can only be contemplated in the presence of complete neurological recovery. This is unlikely in the majority of cases. Therefore *compensated intelligibility* (their italics) is the realistic goal, and strategies of treatment must be directed to making the most of unimpaired function and to utilizing other intact systems. It is not only in relation to the language disability that the patient needs to adjust. He also has to accept that following illness or trauma producing a degree of permanent disablement, life cannot be "the same as before". He must be helped to adapt to a different way of living, and one of the principal aims of any therapist should be that of attempting to ensure that qualitatively this new life is as good as it is possible to make it.

Any rationale of treatment is dependent upon the therapist being able to obtain as much information as possible about the patient. This includes first and foremost a comprehensive medical report, but it may also entail psychologist's and social worker's reports. Treatment will obviously be strongly influenced by knowledge about the likely course of the disease, site of lesion, proposed medication and so forth. In turn, the therapist has an obligation to supply a clear and comprehensive account of the extent of the patient's language disability, together with objectives of treatment to medical advisers and to others concerned with his condition. Preferably of course, such information is better supplemented by verbal discussion but this may not always be possible.

For those patients whose pathological condition predicts a rapid deterioration, as for example in diseases like amyotrophic lateral sclerosis, the therapist adopts a somewhat different role. Long-term goals are patently unrealistic even when these include compensatory measures. On the other hand a complete cessation of intervention may only add to the patient's feelings of depression and rejection. In such cases it is preferable to continue with periodic visits in which general problems relating to speech are discussed and during which such aid as is appropriate can be given. For example, if hand function is reasonable it may be possible to supply one of the small communicators on which the message is "typed" out and displayed either on a printout or a small screen. Treatment is therefore mainly palliative.

A considerable degree of intuitive sensitivity is called for from the clinician in determining when is the best point at which to opt out of treatment. This is particularly necessary when the course of the disease is variable as in conditions like multiple sclerosis. It is important to use remission periods to build up proficiency which will help when there is a further down turn in the course of the condition. As symptoms multiply and exacerbate there will come a time when continuance of therapy will only increase the sense of failure through nonachievement of goals, and tactful withdrawal from active treatment is then the most appropriate action. Quite apart from the specific speech disorder, the general condition of the patient needs to be taken into account when setting objectives of treatment. The onset of dysarthria or dyspraxia is in many cases associated with disease and/or senescent changes where there is a concurrent falling off of other skills. Plainly this will influence one's expectation of success levels. Chronological age in itself is, however, not always a reliable prognostic factor. It needs to be related to other variables such as general motivation and level of support from the patient's family.

Most clinicians can report the paradox of surprisingly successful progress with very elderly patients and a correspondingly disappointing response from much younger people when severity of the condition is not the reason.

Head injured patients form a special category in which the precept of unpredictable progress applies especially.

Age constitutes an additional problem but often it may be one of youthfulness rather than of old age. The resulting extent of impairment from serious brain damage in a young person may be much more traumatic and harder to accept than in an older person who has a background of fulfilment rather than a future of promise. Then too, the type of injury occasioned by the violence say of a road traffic accident may well produce a disorder of affect, of memory and of intellect as well as a specific speech disorder. Goals of recovery are very difficult to determine in such cases since progress is very much subject to the vagaries of the patient's mood, motivation, level of fatigue and intellectual status.

Other conditions which influence prognosis but which may be more readily remedied are hearing loss, visual impairment and dental problems.

Decay in hearing acuity is a well known adjunct of ageing and particular states of pathology may hasten its onset. Loss may be central or peripheral when it may be the outcome of calcification and/or atrophy of auditory structures.

Vision too, may change and in conditions of diffuse neuropathology such as multiple sclerosis, monocular vision or diploplia may be one of the many symptoms.

Balance of tone in the orofacial musculature can change with disease and this is very likely with lower motor neurone involvement which leads to weakness of muscles. Thus, dentures which were previously satisfactory may no longer be retained easily. This can well affect swallowing since normal patterns of deglutition entail occlusion. Case notes frequently mention ill fitting dentures as an additional problem and indeed some patients regard this as the main source of their speech disability!

For children with developmental disorders of speech production aims of therapy have to be evaluated in the context of likely growth and maturation and these natural processes may serve to aid and support remedial work. Fawcus (1971) states that "one of the baffling features of our observation of children whom we would term 'dyspraxic' is the fact that some of them gradually show signs of considerable improvement from what would appear to be a hopeless situation." Maturation could well be one of the factors contributing to the improvement.

It is essential that any linguistic investigation should allow for the normally expected levels of language appropriate for age and intellect. Features characteristic of delay in acquisition of spoken language should be clearly differentiated from those directly attributable to the disorder since it is commonplace in conditions of dysarthria and dyspraxia for both delay and deviance to cooccur.

Children with different types of congenital cerebral pathology will obviously suffer differing degrees of impairment and according to the nature of the condition, salient features of the communication disorder will also differ.

The distribution of spasticity will, for example, influence the severity of the resulting dysarthria. Generally speaking a spastic hemiplegia will not have a *direct* effect on speech production though there may well be associated linguistic problems possibly related to intellectual deficits. A spastic diplegia, however, and to an even greater extent a quadriplegia is likely to result in severe impairment at all levels of the vocal tract so that respiratory, phonatory and articulatory processes will be affected.

The dyskinesia associated with athetoid conditions almost invariably has a grossly deleterious effect on speech production.

Associated Conditions

The presence of associated conditions is an important factor which needs to be borne in mind since these will influence the selection and planning of particular methods of treatment.

Level of intelligence, for example, will influence prognosis in the case of both adults and children. Where this is poor, goals of achievement must necessarily be adjusted. But, a low level of intelligence cannot be assumed purely on the outcome of conventional intelligence tests. Their limitations are too well recognized for such facile conclusions to be drawn.

Reference has been made above to the complicated sequelae of head injury and these will almost certainly affect the outcome of tests. Similarly children with severe physical and linguistic handicap are at a great disadvantage and interpretation of results can be incredibly difficult. Any findings need to be substantiated by evidence from ongoing observation of behaviour.

Level of attention is another aspect likely to influence both assessment and treatment. Ability to attend may deteriorate with the progress of disease, or in developmental conditions it may never reach a mature level. It is recognized that attention changes as a function of maturation progressing from the fleeting stage manifest by the infant through to a fully integrated multichannel stage normally achieved around the age of 5;0–6;0 years. Children with neuromotor disorders may be pathologically distractable. Each and every sound or sight impinging on their environment is accorded equal though momentary attention.

Allied to this distractability are *perceptual difficulties,* particularly of integrating input from different sensory channels. Commonly there is impairment in attending to both auditory and visual stimuli simultaneously; if visual cues are limited then there will be improved auditory attention and vice versa (Edwards, 1973). Extreme cases show complete inability to cross code sensory information resulting in failure to perceive and relate sight with sound or touch. This state amounts to an agnosia. The resulting linguistic disability in developmental conditions is profound and obviously extends well beyond that attributable to the motor dysfunction. However, in milder forms, children with verbal dyspraxia do often demonstrate impairment of perceptual integration. Again assessment of this is difficult since many of the tests require a motor response (e.g. Bender, Gestalt), and where there is a known motor disorder it may not be easy to decide where the impairment lies, whether in the perception or in the execution of the task. Again careful observation will probably yield clues, particularly with regard to the way in which the task is carried out; in the case of drawing figures, for example, a lack of relationship of the different parts to each other may be indicative of perceptual problems.

Depending on the underlying pathology, *epilepsy* may develop and this will influence management programmes. But, there is a need to be alert to the less obvious, insidious onset of petit mal attacks. Any evidence of absence or of undue dreaminess should be carefully noted.

As will be explained in more detail, parents or care-givers have a vital role to play in the rehabilitation programme and to some extent its success is dependent upon their attitude. This can veer between two extremes, the one over caring and over protective and the other, probably for highly complex reasons, rejecting. It is therefore an essential prerequisite of any treatment that time should be spent in explaining, in counselling and in helping towards an acceptance of a realistic prognosis. Until there is such recognition and acceptance, cooperation in rehabilitation cannot be wholly successful.

Investigation and Assessments of Speech

It is apparent therefore that any comprehensive assessment and plan for treatment can only be successfully carried out in the light of full knowledge about all aspects of the patient's function; physical, psychological, social and environmental.

Dysarthria

Objective Assessments

Rosenbek and La Pointe (1978) describe an assessment procedure based on Netsell's 1971 model. This was discussed in Chapter 4. Essentially it entails an evaluation, instrumental where possible, of the 10 functional components or valves which influence aerodynamic forces within the vocal tract. This

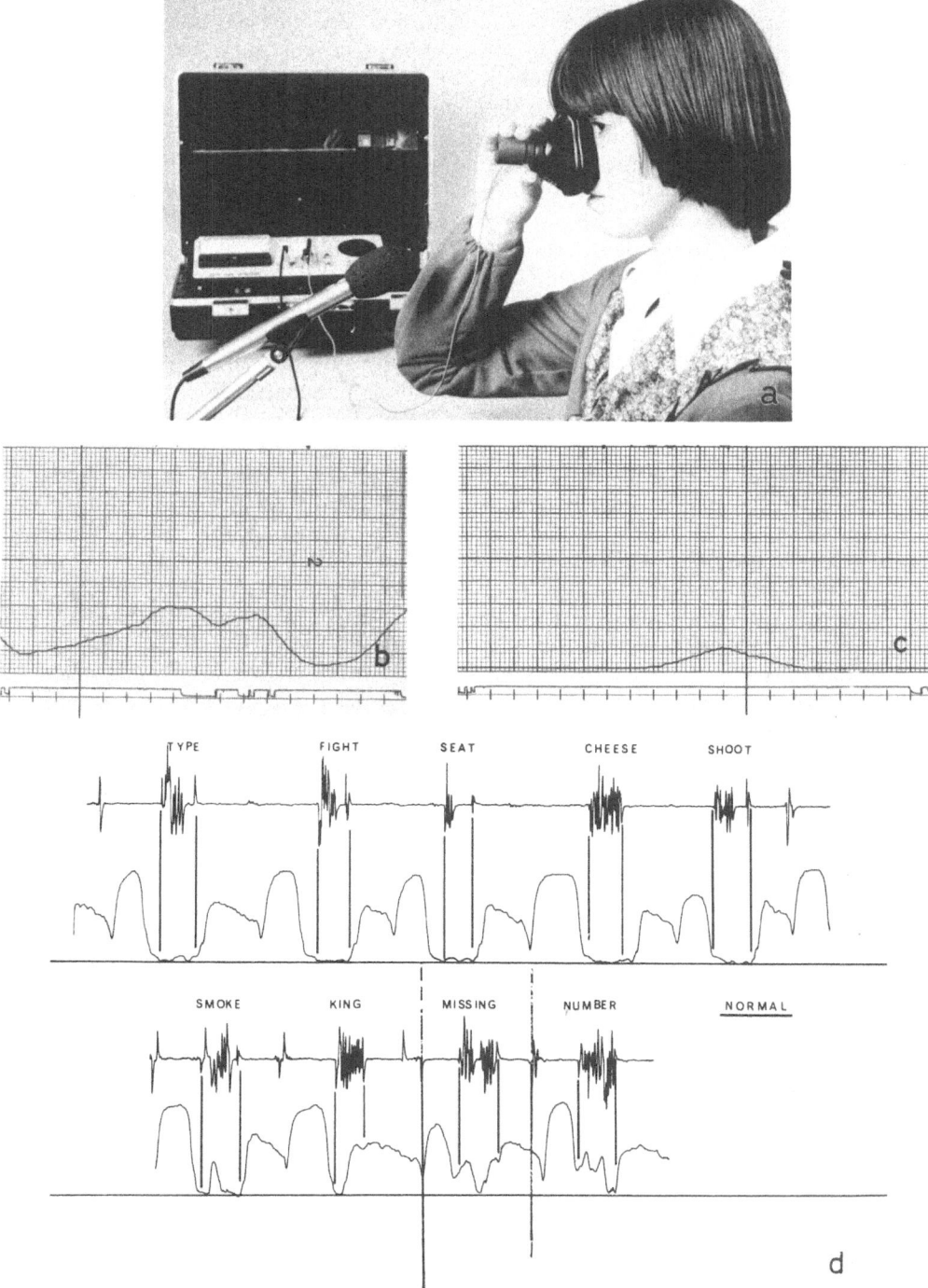

Fig. 17. *a* Nasal anemometer, *b* nasal airflow on production of "missing" before therapy, *c* reduction in nasal airflow after 3 months therapy, *d* anemometer reading of normal production. (Reproduced by permission of R. Ellis and F. Flack and College of Speech Therapists, London)

physiological assessment is complemented by a parallel description of articulation, resonance, phonation, respiration and prosody. The choice of subheadings is certainly open to criticism in that it is questionable whether prosody should be listed separately because of its close relationship with all the other aspects of production. Rosenbek and La Pointe in fact later on make this point themselves but justify inclusion of the parameters on grounds of tradition and on the fact that they provide a convenient framework for diagnosis.

Netsell and Daniel (1979) illustrate the application of the physiological model by reference to a case study of a spastic, flaccid dysarthria subject.

Respiratory components coordinate to ensure adequate subglottal air pressure which acts on the sound source. Degrees of pressure can be measured by use of a water manometer preferably fitted with a bleed valve to ensure that pressure is sustained in holding the level of the water column constant. The authors estimate that ability to generate pressure sufficient to achieve a level of 5–10 cm H_2O over a period of 3–5 seconds is adequate for normal speech.

Laryngeal valving can be measured objectively by use of the laryngograph, Fourcin and Abberton (1971). This provides an ongoing visual record of vocal fold vibration by changes in impedance of an electrical current carried across two electrodes placed one on each side of the thyroid cartilage. The resulting wave form L_x indicates opening and closure phases of the folds. It also indicates some abnormalities of closure.

The velopharyngeal valve is controlled by palatal and pharyngeal musculature. Its efficiency may be assessed by measurement of nasal and oral air flow. The nasal anemometer (Fig. 17a) developed in Exeter by Ellis and Flack (Ellis, 1979) measures nasal air flow. Anthony (1981) has been using pneumotachography to measure differentials of nasal and oral air flow in cases of cleft palate. As yet there is no really totally satisfactory means of measuring nasal resonance. This is because so many factors contribute to it over and above the simple valving action of the velopharynx. (Edwards and Watson, 1981, pp. 91–94).

Fig. 17b, c, d shows readings of nasal air flow. The first, Fig. 17b, demonstrates hypernasality with nasal escape of air on nonnasal sounds. Fig. 17c shows markedly reduced nasality amounting to hyponasal resonance in the same subject. Fig. 17d represents a "normal" reading.

Oral musculature can be assessed by electromyographic (EMG) measurements. Surface electrodes are obviously more convenient to use and are probably adequate provided that measurement of electrical discharge from individual muscle fibres is not critical.

Tongue movement can be estimated by electropalatography (Hardcastle, 1972; Jones, 1977). This is carried out by fitting an acrylic palate carrying 64 electrodes sited in key articulatory contact positions. When the tongue makes contact with one or more of the electrodes, a signal is conducted and converted to a visual display which replicates the shape of the plate. Alternatively the signal may be fed into a computer which samples tongue palate contact at 10 ms intervals. The main disadvantage of this system at present is the need for a purpose-designed palate for each subject but it is hoped that work will proceed on the design of a flexible palate which can be moulded to individual requirements. Work along these lines has been started at the University of Tokyo (Sawashima, 1980), and at the Department of Linguistic Science, Reading University. See Fig. 14, Chapter 5.

A record of aerodynamic function is of considerable value in identifying both level and type of malfunction. Most of the instrumentation described here has the additional advantage of being able to be used for biofeedback techniques in therapy.

Perceptual Assessment

Most workers would supplement such instrumental investigation by perceptual assessment and perhaps in some cases this may still be the only means of evaluation available. It is interesting to note that where objective and perceptual investigations have been carried out in parallel, in broad respects, there is accord in evaluation, but it is in the identification of fine detail contributing to the overall pattern that objective measurement is superior.

Whereas, it is obviously preferable in the interests of good treatment programmes that both types of investigation should be undertaken, real life situations may find the therapist without such facilities.

In these circumstances it is perfectly possible to derive a reasonable amount of information about vocal tract function through assessment of each of the components or subsystems contributing to speech production, *respiration* being logically the first.

Adequate control of the egressive air stream is likely to present a much greater barrier to phonation than reduced pulmonary air capacity. The tidal volume required for speech represents only about 25% of the total vital capacity. Intensity, that is, volume, may be diminished if there is restriction of thoracic movement as this will reduce the pressure of the ascending subglottic air column, but the controlled expiration of air is far more likely to be difficult.

Phonation will be affected by excess breathy quality and because of air wastage speech may consist largely of short sentences or phrases, often syntactically incomplete.

Assessment of breathing should be related to speech. Counting, repetitions of strings of consonant-vowel (CV) syllables, various forms of serial speech will provide impressionistic information about volume and control of expiration, and its effect upon speech. Coordination of diaphragmatic, costal and abdominal movement should be noted.

There is considerable confusion of terminology in descriptions of abnormal *phonation* and it is often unclear as to what is meant by such terms as *strained* and *strangled*. Is one a more severe form of the other? Similarly *wet, hoarse* etc.: seem equally opaque terms. One of the more recent subjective assessments is that produced by Laver (1980b). It takes as its starting point a hypothesized neutral state of the vocal tract and describes in phonetic terms different voice types which depart from this setting. Even so it is still difficult to be precise in identifying the different parameters and the analysis entails a training period as a necessary measure towards ensuring interlistener agreement.

8*

Laryngeal activity is of course interrelated with respiration (see above) and phonatory disorder can equally be due to aberrant expiratory patterns contributing to irregularities of vocal fold function, as much as to dysfunction of the folds themselves. Similarly the cause may lie in abnormalities of extrinsic laryngeal muscle movement, resulting in changes in laryngeal position and affecting tension and closure of the vocal folds. Excess tension may produce abnormal pitch with very narrow variation. Phonological and phonetic interpretations of pitch, and intonation have been discussed previously; in this particular context the reference is to motor correlates of pitch. Voicing onset time (VOT) has also been discussed in relation to phonological and phonetic aspects and any difficulties in signalling contrasts between voiced sounds and their voiceless cognates should be noted.

Stress is related to intensity and timing of the expiratory air stream.

Any assessment of prosody therefore needs to take into consideration function throughout the entire vocal tract. The possiblity of an underlying linguistic rather than a motor disability or indeed the coexistence of both must be borne in mind.

It is notoriously difficult to specify a clear division between *phonation* and *resonance* but in the present context, the term is confined to *nasal* resonance. There is evidence that compensatory efforts to minimize hypernasal resonance may lead to abnormal phonation through raising of the larynx.

Disorders of resonance may also be associated with other vocal tract dysfunction as part of a neurological disorder (cf. motor neurone disease). Of all the parameters of speech production nasal resonance is probably the most elusive to define subjectively. This is for a number of reasons, but the principal one is that because there is such a wide band of variation in what constitutes "normal nasal resonance" there is a corresponding variation in listener evaluation. Informal studies have demonstrated that even among trained listeners, a consensus of view is difficult to achieve. Fletcher (1978) commenting on the problem of perceptual evaluation advocates instrumental measurement with the use of the TONAR which is a device developed by him yielding a ratio measurement between nasal and oral air pressure in speech.

Visual examination of the velopharyngeal port is also unreliable without recourse to instrumentation since much of its effectiveness is due to movement above the level of the soft palate and therefore not visible on oral inspection, in particular the lateral excursion of the naso- and oropharyngeal walls. Another factor to be considered is that velopharyngeal movement is not an on-off phenomenon. In the first place there is a marked difference between movement for speech and for non speech. There is also considerable variation between different sounds in speech. Movement is greater for obstruent sounds (stops, fricatives and affricates) and for high vowels. Dickson and Maue–Dickson (1982) note that the action of the walls of the naso- and oropharynx bear an inverse relationship to each other. Context of the utterance will also influence the extent of movement.

Hypernasal resonance is also the outcome of conditions other than primary velopharyngeal incompetence. Abnormal tongue posture where the back of the tongue is retracted will increase nasality as will also the relationship of upper and lower jaw; a narrow opening tending to increase nasality.

Articulation

Evaluation of movement of the articulators in a nonspeech context is of dubious value and really tells one little about the patient's true capacity for speech. Of greater importance is an assessment of the degree of retention or the potential for development of a motor *equivalent* representation of the required utterance. For example, tongue protrusion is often included as a part of the battery of assessment of articulation, yet no English sound calls for this movement.

Overall intelligibility is a much more useful concept. A recent assessment published by Yorkston and Beukelman (1981) provides a measure of intelligibility and speaking rate. The authors claim that this serves to grade different dysarthric speakers, to make comparisons with normal speech and to monitor change. The patient is assessed on single word, and on sentence intelligibility as well as on overall rate of speech. From this data a communication efficiency ratio is derived through comparison of the rate of intelligible speech produced by the dysarthric speaker with the mean rate of intelligible speech produced by a group of normal speakers. Norms are obtained for 20 speakers, but ages are not specified. There is evidence that rate of speech slows as a function of normal ageing processes (Ryan, 1972; Ryan and Burk, 1974). The age factor should therefore be taken into account in any assessment of elderly patients.

For more detailed information about the patient's phonological system and phonetic realizations it is desirable that some analysis should be made of ongoing speech.

Enderby (1980, 1983) has developed a standardized profile which rates efficiency at different points along the vocal tract through performance on tasks some of which involve speech. Results are scored on a 9-point scale. Additionally reflex' activity (coughing, swallow, dribble) and overall intelligibility are rated. The assessment was standardized on two groups of normal speakers age range 23–64 and 60–97. No significant difference in performance emerged between the two groups. However, this similarity may have arisen in part from placing too low a ceiling for some of the tasks; at upper levels of performance differences might have been observed particularly in relation to timing. The evidence of many other studies on speech changes in the elderly would tend to substantiate this view (for a review see Mitchell in Edwards, 1982b). Using the format of the profile Enderby (1983) has analysed features of dysarthria and has produced characteristic profiles for the main types of dysarthria based on underlying neurological conditions. As a starting point and for the purpose of transmitting clinical data to other professionals these profiles are valuable. But as their author would no doubt agree, for the Speech Therapist undertaking treatment, they serve principally to indicate the features of the dysarthria which will require subsequent investigation in much greater detail.

Linguistic Investigation

It is essential that phonological analysis of segmental and nonsegmental features be undertaken and indeed this analysis should extend to other levels of language too.

Unlike dyspraxic subjects, those who are dysarthric show a measure of consistency in error pattern. There are several articulatory assessments which may be used; most of these rely upon elicited response to pictures or objects. This, while being an expedient way of transcribing utterance tends to give an enhanced picture, in so far as performance on a one-word off basis will probably be very different from that in continuous speech. Another limitation of standardized tests is that many are limited to consonant systems and this is unfortunate since analysis of vowel systems yields valuable information about timing aspects of production as well as about resonance and phonation. Probably the most representative sample can be obtained by a high quality audiorecording of a stretch of speech. Crystal (1983) has published profiles which extend an earlier procedure concerned with syntactic screening (Crystal, Fletcher and Garman, 1976, 1982). These are concerned with the profiling of phonology (PROPH), prosody (PROP) and semantics (PRISM).

The phonological profile starting from a data base of phonetically transcribed utterances proceeds to a classification of the subject's sound system both in terms of distribution within syllables and phonetic type according to manner and place of production. There is also provision for analysis of vowels. A number of options are then available for further interpretation of the data so that for remedial purposes patterns of deviance may be described. While it is recognized that phonetic errors will preponderate in cases of dysarthria, this phonological profile nevertheless provides a useful framework in which to identify error patterns.

The same conditions apply to the prosodic profile. This is mainly concerned with intonation, but the notation relevant to linguistic prosody, that is tone, tonicity etc., is also a convenient way of noting motor disability.

Such a method of data collection is time consuming insofar as it calls for painstaking transcription but the value of the results as it relates to subsequent planning of treatment more than compensates for this. As Crystal (1982) writes: "To know that in 10 minutes (of sampling time) *everything* the patient did linguistically is down on paper provides an empirical datum whose value cannot be underestimated. Transcription time is time well spent. On it the whole basis of one's analytical edifice stands."

Dyspraxia

Dyspraxia does not lend itself so readily to instrumental investigation for assessment and one is therefore more reliant on the "empirical datum" of linguistic information together with evidence of eyes and ears about the general behaviour of the patient. Quantity of data is therefore an important factor. Audiorecordings are useful but they offer an incomplete account unless accompanied by detailed notes. They do not stand comparison with videorecordings.

A visual representation enables the viewer subsequently to spot subtle nuances of behaviour, as for example, the almost imperceptible shift of organs of articulation in one direction before changing to another in the quest for the correct placement. Fleeting movements of lips and tongue may be observed confirming a last second change from one sound to another.

Any assessment as well as including samples of speech, both spontaneous and in performance of set tasks, should also include data on *nonspeech behaviour*. Gross and fine motor movements, performance of rhythmic sequences; all these should be recorded. Gordon and McKinley (1980) decribe a very simple screening test for assessment of motor control. This is the "coffee jar test" and it provides a quick and useful means of gauging initially the extent of motor disability so that further more detailed investigation can be undertaken as and if appropriate. The test includes assessment of balance and coordination and locomotor skill, through tasks such as walking along a line heel to toe, threading beads, unscrewing lids, drawing and copying shapes. Edwards (1982a) used the protocol listed in Table 2 as a guide in the assessment of children referred as possible dyspraxics.

These tasks when possible were carried out with an accompanying videorecording which could subsequently be assessed.

Data obtained from these assessments have been described in some detail in Chapter 5. The spontaneous language samples taken in conjunction with test items were most valuable in confirming characteristic errors.

Macaluso Haynes (1978) bases therapy for dyspraxia of speech very much along sensory motor principles. This is in accord with Berry (1980) who relates certain types of articulatory errors to faulty auditory haptic integration. This term refers to the ability to code information across sensory channels; in this case to relate sounds heard to the appropriate oral movements associated with their production. Oral perception is, however, exceedingly elusive to evaluate. The author used an oral stereognostic recognition task employing various shapes and textures in a survey of children with articulatory defects associated with cleft palate (Edwards, 1981). But the results while demonstrating inferior skills in the children when compared with controls were not on the whole very satisfactory since at the most it could only be claimed that they measured a mix of tactile and kinaesthetic perception. Furthermore, as the shapes had to be manipulated by the tongue there was also a strong motor element.

Diadochokinetic tests appear to differentiate dyspraxic children from those with functional types of disorder. In fact, most of the children diagnosed as dyspraxic fall well below the norms suggested by Canning and Rose (1974) for performance of these tasks. Fletcher (1978) has published a diadochokinetic rate scale. This rates speed of movement in repetition of nonsense syllables. The test provides norms for ages 6;0–13;0. It does not include any qualitative measurement of performance.

Syllable rate is also included in Blakely's (1980) screening test for Developmental Apraxia of Speech. There are eight subtests, the first being a measure of expressive language discrepancy.

Table 2. *Assessment of verbal dyspraxia*

1. Sample of spontaneous speech – video recorded.

2. Tongue movement a) Imitated b) Command c) Sequential.
   Up Down Out In Circular No. correct: No. groping/incorrect:
                                    a)
                                    b)
                                    c)
   Up and Down. Out-Circular-In.

3. Lip movment a) Imitated b) Command.
   Smile. Pout. Blow. No. correct: No. groping/incorrect:

4. Sounds in isolation. Transcribe: "Say these sounds after me:"
   p b t d s z ch j
   st   sk   sm
   kl   kr   kw
   fl   fr
   bl   br   pl   pr

5. Imitation of words. Transcribe. "I want you to say this word three times. I'll say it first and then you say it."
   Repeat each word three times. Repeat stimulus if necessary.

cat	basket	television
door	sticky	vegetables
baby	television	communicate
patacake	canary	particular
	stocking	caterpillar

6. Imitation of short phrases. Mark stress and intonation: "I want you to say exactly what I say. I'll say it first, then you." (Repeat if necessary.)

   A cup of coffee please!

   Can you catch the ball?

   The tractor went *crash* into the red car.
   The *tractor* went crash into the red car.
   The tractor went crash into the *red* car.

   I like treacle toffee.
   I *like* treacle toffee.
   I like *treacle* toffee.

7. Rapid Alternating Movement. Establish each sound in isolation and then in sequence before starting timing.
   p t k   speed in secs/10 repetitions (Refer. Canning and Rose, 1974 for norms)
   buttercup

8. Imitation of clapping rhythms   – = stressed clap
   – –   / = unstressed clap
   – / –
   / / – –
   / – – / /

9. Gross motor movement – videotape
   hopping on each foot
   jumping
   catching
   throwing   No. correct:

10. Sample of drawing, e.g. man, house, clock.

11. Sample of writing, copying, spontaneous   } where appropriate

12. Sample of reading aloud (recorded)

Many studies have demonstrated an imbalance between levels of language comprehension and expression, with the former being superior to the latter in developmental verbal dyspraxia, but as was indicated in Chapter 4 this may be apparent rather than real. Blakely's screening test relies on somewhat tenuous data to arrive at this discrepancy score. It is suggested that comprehension be assessed by the Peabody Picture Vocabulatory Test (PPVT). Both this and the British version, the EPVT, really only evaluate lexical items. They give little information about syntactic or semantic aspects. The choice of test for measurement of expressive language is left to the examiner. Mean length of utterance is one measure suggested. For each test a language age is recorded. This is a notoriously unreliable representation since the language age rarely is a true reflection of the chronological stage it purports to represent. A child of six with a reported language age of three years will not talk as a three year old. Some aspects of his language may be below the level, others above.

The other subtests record performance on vowels and diphthongs, oral motor movement verbal sequencing, articulation, motorically complex words transpositions and prosody. The last item is subjectively assessed on a three point scale. This assessment provides a useful format for assessment of dyspraxia but to assign significance to a final score is probably not very fruitful if the language discrepancy score is included. Norms are printed for the other subtests and individual comparisons can be made with them.

Rosenbek (1978) has described fully the assessment of dyspraxia he and Wertz have developed. This takes the Mayo model as a starting point but it moves towards a considerably less narrow interpretation of the condition as a pure motor disorder. By acknowledging dysprosody as an intrinsic feature it gives recognition to the nonsegmental aspects of the disorder.

Some of the standard tests normally used in assessment of aphasia also include sections which evaluate apraxia. It is claimed for example that the Porch Index of Communicative Ability (PICA, 1967) reveals a typical profile for dyspraxic subjects but this really tells one very little about the nature of the linguistic disorder.

The Boston Diagnostic Aphasia Examination (BDAE, 1972) also assesses phonemic errors and prosodic disability albeit in a fairly cursory manner, but in line with a Geschwindian model interprets these errors as evidence of disconnection and assigns them to aphasic classifications.

Intervention

Setting and Frequency

The majority of adults are seen in hospital clinics or in rehabilitation units. There are both advantages and disadvantages to this practice. In favour is the availability of more sophisticated equipment for treatment which can be located in one centre with the necessary technical support at hand to ensure its optimum use. Against, is the inevitability of long fatiguing hours spent in ambulances en route to the centre. The patient is also seen in an artificial environment which is not ideal for the promotion of functional communication and special efforts have to be made to establish contact with relatives. Day hospitals to some extent overcome the fatigue factor in that attendance covers a longer span of time. However, at the present time in most places, patients can only attend these if they have additional physical disability.

Most clinicians agree that frequent treatment is beneficial for both adults and children particularly in the early stages. There do not as yet appear to have been any well designed studies which either support or refute this belief. But since one of the main thrusts of therapy is the establishment and generalization of new techniques of communication these are more likely to be fostered through frequent monitoring and reinforcement on the part of the therapist. Obviously much will depend upon the nature of the patient's condition. Such a rigorous regime for those suffering from debilitating illnesses like myasthenia gravis would be strongly contraindicated.

Flexibility in determining frequency of therapy is probably the best counsel. Few therapists now look upon therapy as being continuous on a once-weekly basis. By evaluating rate of progress it is advantageous to vary the regime by providing intensive therapy when motivation is high and progress may be predicted, while slowing down the pace when the patient is less fit. Breaks in therapy followed by booster sessions often produce more positive results than a similar number of sessions running consecutively. Children require somewhat different conditions and frequency of treatment is closely linked to the setting in which the child can be seen and also the availability of parents to ensure frequent attendance and to provide support.

If the language disability is part of a much wider handicap as is often the case in dysarthria, it is likely that such children will be seen in a school or nursery unit. This offers the opportunity for frequent therapy and also for inculcating techniques learned, into the context of general educational programmes. Here too, there is often a good opportunity for working cooperatively with other remedial therapists as well as with teachers and nursery assistants. Ideally the parent(s) should be equally involved but practicalities often make this difficult to achieve. Therefore additional efforts must be made to ensure that they are fully informed about the aims of therapy as well as being shown the ways in which it is hoped to achieve these.

In recent years there has been a marked trend towards the greater *active* involvement of parents or caregivers in their childrens' rehabilitation programmes. This amounts to far more than the parent sitting in on the treatment session. It entails detailed preparation of joint programmes on the part of the therapist, the demonstration of these and the monitoring of their execution. From anecdotal evidence it appears likely that parents who participate to this extent in remediation place much higher value on the successful outcome of therapy.

Such procedures need to be supported by explanatory sessions possibly through group meetings of parents. The fact that "professionals tell their patients nothing" is a well worn cliché, but also unfortunately in many cases a true one. Understanding the nature of the communicative disability is undoubtedly in some measure a help towards its remedy.

Most children with a severe degree of handicap are likely to find themselves attending a special centre; for very young children this may be one which is neurologically orientated. The great advantage of such a setting is the assurance of thorough investigation by a team of workers of all facets of the child's condition and behaviour, as well as the opportunity provided for joint programmes. This type of intervention is well described by Gordon and McKinlay (1980) where the needs of clumsy children are discussed. There is a growing number of such centres throughout the United Kingdom, and implementation of the recommendations of the Court report (1979) should ensure a more cooperative approach to the problems of such children with multiple handicaps. The 1981 Education Act provides specifically for children with special needs, that is to say those with various types of handicap. As an aftermath of the earlier Warnock Report it recommends that wherever possible children who require special educational provision should receive this in an environment alongside nonhandicapped children. In the case of children with language disability, in many cases, this practice has distinct advantages since it thereby allows for such children to mix with normally speaking peer groups who can provide appropriate models of speech production. Again, extra care must be taken to ensure that parents are brought into the programme as active participants and not just as passive observers.

Groups Versus Individual Therapy

Of course, this is not an either/or situation. Some patients benefit from both types of intervention taking place concurrently since each provides a slightly different focus on the language disorder. Nevertheless, a group is more than a heterogenous collection of people brought together because of one common condition. Abercrombie's (1960) experience of setting up tutorial groups for medical students contains much sound advice which may be applied to remedial settings. It is also important at the outset to determine what the aims of the group are. Is it to reinforce techniques previously learned in individual therapy, or is it, for example, to foster psychosocial skills and to build up the patient's confidence and his ability to communicate? The last few years have seen a proliferation of literature describing these aspects of behaviour. Hargie Saunders and Dickson (1981) is one of the readable texts which discusses interpersonal communication.

Early stages of treatment will probably need to be carried out on a one-to-one basis for it is only in this way that the patient can learn to develop his own particular strengths and adopt compensatory measures for weaknesses.

Recently there is a growing tendency towards the organization of specific intensive courses for people with particular types of disorder. Such courses have long been established for stammerers, but it is only in the past year that patients with Parkinson's disease have been offered a similar type of course. This was initiated in 1981 with the help of the Parkinson Disease Society and will be reported (Robertson forthcoming). It has been repeated in Nottingham in 1982 (Chipperfield and Berman, unpublished). 10 patients attended this residential course over a period of 14 days. They reflected different levels of disability; all were on medication and some had also undergone surgery. Mornings were spent in carrying out intensive speech programmes both individually and in groups while in the afternoon there was a choice between leisure activities (outings and trips to various places) or more speech therapy. Early results are encouraging, particularly in relation to gains in individual cases, but one of the difficulties is the need to maintain progress when they return home, particularly in the case of those for whom no speech therapy is available. An evaluation can only be made in the light of sustained gains. This type of therapy, however, is valuable in increasing motivation and in providing opportunity for reinforcement. Its extension to other types of disorder is well worth considering. A further projected study (Robertson and Thompson) addresses the question of maintenance of gains over a longer period.

Multidisciplinary Involvement

Since in many cases the communication disorder is one among many other handicaps, rehabilitation practice in recent years has concentrated increasingly on the need for a multidisciplinary approach to the patient. This has merit in that it avoids overlap of similar techniques and provides for the utilization of therapy carried out by allied disciplines. This type of intervention may best be illustrated by the recommendations of a study group conducted by Trent Regional Health Authority (1982) in which members of the remedial professions (physiotherapy, occupational therapy and speech therapy) took part. The medical consultant presented the initial case history and in the final session, when recommendations were made, the patient was also present to comment on these.

In this particular instance, the patient was a girl aged 19 who had sustained widerspread brain damage following anaesthetic failure, while undergoing an appendectomy, during vacation overseas. Prior to this accident she had been preparing to enter University to study Biochemistry.

The participants were required to plan in outline a remedial programme based on interdisciplinary therapy. Following individual assessments, they suggested group discussion, during which they would attempt to gain overall knowledge of the patient's capabilities and to determine in the long term, likely level of recovery. The emphasis was very much on seeing the patient as a whole person not as a conglomerate of various handicaps. Short-term aims were considered from the point of active cooperation between different professions for some aspects of remediation. It was thought, for example, that occupational therapists and nursing staff would work together in helping the patient to learn to dress herself, physiotherapists and speech therapists would combine on work relating to respiration and phonation, and so on. The social worker would provide the interface between the patient's home and the rehabilitation centre and would be a key figure in helping parents or spouses (in this particular case a widowed mother), towards an understanding both of the extent of the patient's handicap and of her potential for recovery. The expectations of the entire team would be influenced by the clinical psychologist's findings on intellectual status and on personality.

This interdisciplinary programme stressed throughout the importance of functional therapy, that is, remedial work related directly to real life situations.

In fact, at the time of this study group, nearly two years after the initial trauma and a great amount of therapy, the patient has made a good recovery. She is likely to remain wheelchair bound, but she now has reasonable use of her hands and is learning to type. Her speech from a condition of anarthria is at the present time characteristic of a cerebellar type dysarthria. Articulation is clear, but prosody in relation to timing, rate and intonation is the predominant feature of disorder. Motivation from being very poor indeed has improved, though there remains a fair degree of passivity interspersed with bouts of depression about her future. This is now being given active consideration and it is hoped that she may soon embark on a programme of further education, though this may not as yet be at University level.

The value of such a programme of intervention in similar cases cannot be overstated since the effect of a combined coordinated approach far exceeds the sum of the efforts of individual therapies.

Treatment Procedures

Luria (1970) described a regime of therapy based on what he termed intersystemic and intrasystemic reorganization. The former relies on the development of other skills as an aid to promoting communicative ability. Use of self-generated rhythm, for example, as in tapping out rhythms is one instance of intersystemic strategy. Interestingly Deal and Darley found that an *externally* imposed rhythm as in using a metronome made little difference to fluency. Writing with speaking is another intersystemic method. Intrasystemic organization involves utilizing lower, more automatic levels of behaviour to facilitate purposive action. This is particularly applicable in remedial work for dyspraxia where these may be relatively intact. It is aimed particularly at phonological reorganization. For example, it is suggested that tongue protrusion may be utilized to develop use of /Θ/ and blowing will encourage plosive sounds. This appears to offer an approach which may only be useful for very severely handicapped people. Certainly it is in direct contradiction to the principles of intervention advocated as a result of the models described throughout this text.

Welford (1979) endorses this view when he states: "... when we speak of 'movements' we need to bear clearly in mind that we are not primarily concerned with patterns of muscular contraction but with something more central and less tangible which has to do with the choosing, programming and controlling of action in order to match achievement to aim." In relation to speech this means that achievement should be demonstrated by coordinated, coherent production in accordance with the initial planning of the utterance. For this to take place, features of allophonic variation, of changing length and stress have to be accounted for. Production of intelligible speech entails far more than the stringing together of separate articulatory segments.

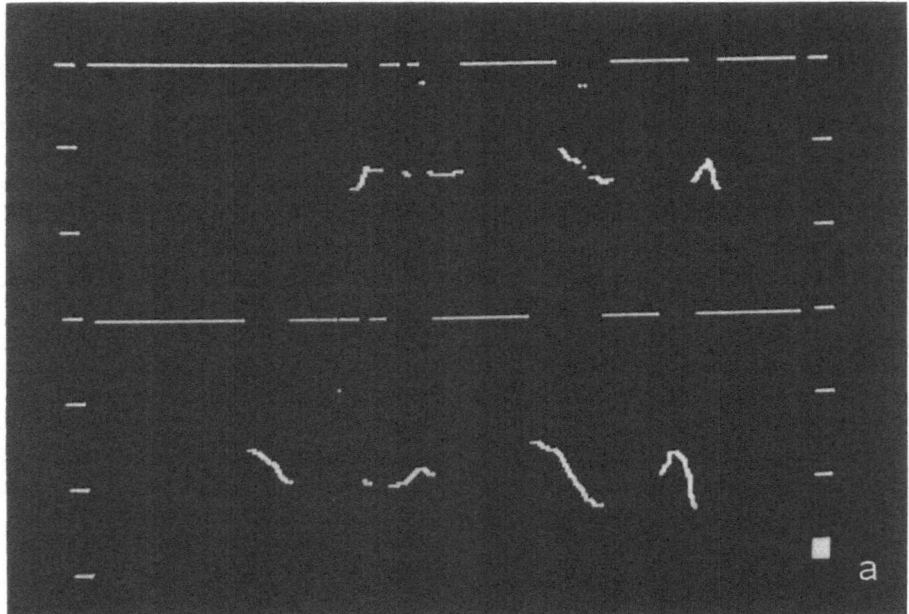

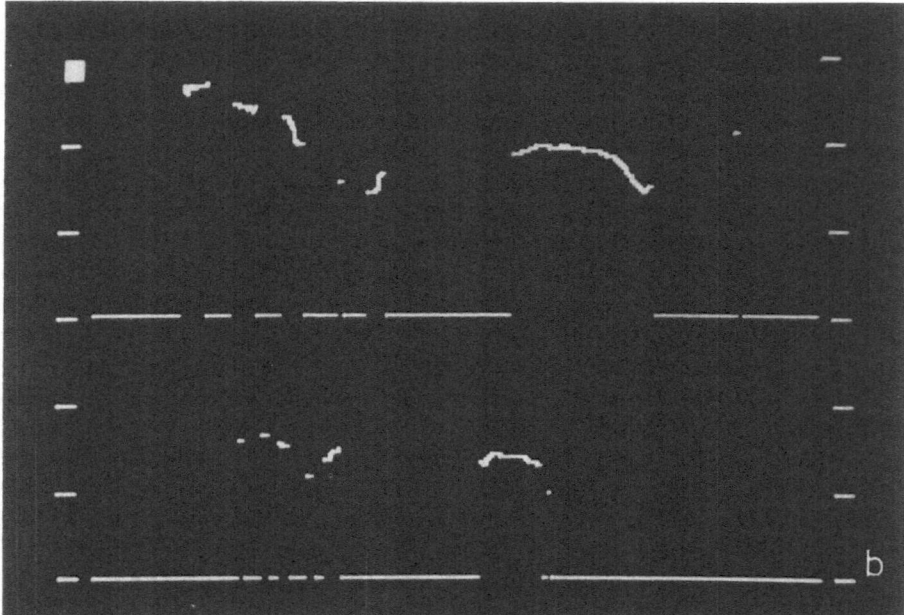

Fig. 18a and b. Intonation patterns demonstrated on visispeech. Patient aged 67 with Parkinson's disease of 3½ years standing, currently on medication. Speech is the most severe presenting symptom. Upper trace represents model. Lower trace represents patient's attempt to imitate. 18a. *Hello, How are you?* 18b. *Are you staying at home for Christmas or are you going away?* Note. 18a. Extraneous initial fall of pitch prior to initiation of utterance, also exaggerated swing between high and low pitch. 18b. Longer phrase, shows compression of overall pattern due to increase in speed of utterance

Therapy is based on a number of different procedures. One of the most successful appears to be that incorporating principles of *biofeedback*.

Having established the particular level of production on which work should start, the patient is given feedback to help him to monitor progress in acquiring the necessary skill.

The Visispeech developed by the Royal National Institute for the Deaf and Jessop Electrics is a particularly useful example. It displays on a TV screen, intonation and stress patterns generated by the speaker. The therapist is able to provide the model and subsequent attempts are recorded and compared. Linked to a computer it is able to sample speech at regular intervals and to store data as well as providing a print out. Successful work has also been undertaken with the laryngograph (voicescope) developed by Fourcin and Abberton (1971). Originally intended for deaf speakers it has proved valuable in providing visual feedback in cases of dysphonia and prosodic disorder. Such devices have greatly aided the work of the therapist by introducing a third sensory channel additional to auditory and kinaesthetic in the modification of speech production.

Netsell and Daniel (1979) provide an excellent example of a rehabilitation programme undertaken with a road traffic accident victim which was based on different types of feedback.

Another type is the visible speech aid devised by Tudor and Selly (1974). This appliance consists of an acrylic palate, the posterior edge of which is fitted with two embedded electrodes which are connected to a control box. When the palate is at rest a current passes through and a light shows in the control box. On elevation of the palate this is extinguished. However, this only responds for anterio-posterior movement of the velum and does not register lateral pharyngeal movement which also contributes to resonance.

Devices which alter production are also thought to be useful. Downie Low and Lindsey (1981) have reported on the use of a delayed auditory feedback (DAF) device with Parkinson patients. This appears to be most useful in controlling rate of production. They found a delay of about 50 ms produced the best results. The device did not prove helpful where there was a reduction in speed of production. Rosenbek and La Pointe (1978) also report the use of DAF and they extend it to other types of dysarthria, but observe that flaccid dysarthria does not respond. They also note that the delay time is critical; too long a delay may have a deleterious effect on production.

A more readily available device is a pacing board described by Helm. This is useful in all cases where timing is one of the problems. The patient taps out the rhythm of the message synchronously with the verbal counterpart.

Noninstrumental procedures include Melodic Intonation Therapy (Sparks, Helm and Albert, 1974). This system was originally developed as a method of aphasia rehabilitation and is based on a postulated theory of right hemisphere dominance for music (for counter arguments see Chapter 2, page 10). The patient is required to learn the intoning of propositional sentences in a manner which replicates the natural prosody of the sentence, if it were spoken. It has been used with dyspraxic patients and some success has been reported. This could be the result of providing a strong rhythmic framework. A similar result might be obtained if this method were used with accelerated types of dysarthria.

Amplification may be used both as a palliative and therapeutic measure. A number of commercial amplifiers are available and these are described in some detail through the text of Greene (1980).

Orosensory stimulation has also been used as a treatment procedure, particularly with apraxic cases. Macaluso Haynes (1978) describes a successful treatment regime based on intensive orosensory therapy with a late adolescent boy whose developmental dyspraxia had proved intransigent to all previous methods of intervention. It is very possible that not all types of dyspraxia would respond to this method of treatment and it would be interesting to try to establish whether there is a differential response between those with predominantly phonological as against phonetic impairment.

Techniques of proprioceptive neuromuscular facilitation and Brushing and Icing have been used with both dysarthric and dyspraxic patients. However, it appears that PNF is only effective where there is peripheral weakness. Its value is therefore questionable in the case of upper motor neurone lesions and for dyspraxia.

Caution also needs to be exercised in the use of icing techniques. Excess may exacerbate the condition it is designed to relieve. Physiotherapists have reported (anecdotal) evidence of impairment of fine motor coordination of hand movements and also signs of slurred speech following prolonged handling of ice in therapy.

Treatment of children with verbal dyspraxia may conveniently be summarized in the following way:

Principles − *Establish* −

- a differentiation between deviance which is specific and that which is concurrent, e.g. features of delay;
- differentiation between disorders of phonetic and phonological origin;
  the degree of overall motor coordination;
  the level(s) of difficulty and determine priorities;
  the level of comprehension;
  the level of intelligence;
  the level of attention;
  the level of monitoring skill;
  a realistic expectation of goals which may be achieved.

Strategies

Provision of a defined rhythmic foundation of which language production becomes an integral part.
Maximization of alternative methods, i.e. intersystemic reorganization through, e.g. writing, visual sequencing, oral awareness, reading.
Development of joint programmes with other workers where appropriate.

Levels of work

respiration,
development of sequences of coordinated rhythmic movement,

oral awareness,
nonsegmental: intonation, stress, rhythm, timing, pause,
sequencing of sounds,
increasing syntactic complexity appropriate to age and developmental
status.

A number of programmes of work have recently been developed for use
with dysarthric and dyspraxic patients.

These can be extremely useful adjuncts to other work with patients
provided that they are adapted to the therapist's principles and strategies of
treatment which have evolved in the light of a particular patient's needs. They
are not intended to offer a "cook book" approach to remediation. The
previous section describing a multidisciplinary programme is a fitting
illustration of the need for individually designed programmes of work.

Reference has already been made to team work and while this is a
currently "vogue term", it is particularly apposite to the conditions which have
been described throughout the book. Rarely do they occur as isolated
disorders of speech. Emphasis has been laid upon the programming and
planning of movement and upon its synergistic aspects. Similar disorders
underlie other aspects of behaviour and physiotherapists are, for example, in a
specially favourable position to help the speech therapist in the establishment
or relearning of coordinated movement. Kimura, for example, regards verbal
dyspraxia as simply one facet of disordered movement and not as a specifically
linguistic disorder (Kimura and Archbold, 1974). Though this view is flawed in
that is does not account for many linguistic-specific features, what is important
is, that though differences exist, so do similarities in the planning and control
of motor activity. The concept of motor equivalence, for example, is not
peculiar to speech.

Where the disorder is of such severity that it is necessary to teach
individual sounds is it good policy to be attempting to teach the patient spoken
language at all? Might not one of the nonverbal systems be more appropriate
either by signing or recourse to one of the increasing number of instrumental
aids.

For patients who can never be expected to achieve intelligible speech, a
whole new vista is now beginning to appear. Currently under development is a
wide range of aids designed to provide an alternative form of communication.
These rely on visual display and in some cases on synthetic speech.
Undoubtedly the next few years will see considerable advancement in the
development of these aids. The present government in the United Kingdom in
conjunction with the Royal Association for Disablement and Rehabilitation
(RADAR) has sponsored a number of centres where patients will be able to
sample different types of aids and where research on the efficacy of existing
instrumentation together with assessment of new devices may be carried out.
For those concerned with facilitating communication this is a most exciting
prospect. Whereas in the past there has been a tremendous obligation to
attempt to achieve speech at all costs and at whatever level of intelligibility,
because alternatives where few and for the most part unsatisfactory, the

opportunity offered by new electronic aids enables the therapist to focus work on making the patient adept in their use and thus providing him with a far more effective method of communication. The development of appropriate computer programs is a fruitful area for research.

It will be noticed that paradoxically in a text purporting to describe disorders of articulation little emphasis is laid on articulatory drills as a treatment procedure. This is deliberate as it is felt that such practice contributes minimally to the patient's recovery.

Far more important than articulation is the concentration on development of synergies of movement for speech and on improving prosodic features. It is these which confer intelligibility. Articulation has its place only as part of the fabric of speech production. As such it cannot be regarded as a separate entity, but must be seen as one component of complete communication verbal and nonverbal.

References

Abbs, J. H. (1973): The influence of the gamma motor system on jaw movements during speech. J. Sp. Hear. Res. *16,* 175–200.

Abbs, J. H. (1979): Speech Motor Equivalence: the need for a multi level control mode. In: Proceedings of 9th Int. Nat. Congr. Phonetic Sciences, Copenhagen, Institute of Phonetics.

Abercrombie, M. L. J. (1960): The Anatomy of Judgement. London: Hutchinson.

Allen, C. M., Turner, J. W., Gadea Cirea, M. (1966): Investigations into speech disturbances following stereotaxic surgery for Parkinsonism. Brit. J. Dis. Comm. *1,* 1, 55–59.

Allen, G. I., Korn, H., Oshima, T., Toyama, K. (1975): The mode of synaptic linkage in the cerebro-ponto-cerebellar pathway of the cat. 11. Responses of single cells in the pontine nuclei. Exp. Brain Res. *24,* 15–36.

Anthony, J. F. K. (1981): Aerodynamic and phonetic analysis. In: Advances in the Management of Cleft Palate (Edwards, M., Watson, A., eds.). Edinburgh: Churchill Livingstone.

Arbib, M. A. (1980): Interacting schemas for motor control. In: Tutorials in Motor Behavior (Stelmach, G. E., Requin, J., eds.). Amsterdam: North-Holland.

Arbib, M. A. (1981): Perceptual structures and distributed motor control. In: Handbook of Physiology Vol. III (Brooks, V. B., ed.). Bethesda, Md.: American Physiological Society.

Barr, M. L. (1979): The Human Nervous System, 3rd ed. New York: Harper & Row.

Bell, D. S. (1968): Speech functions of the thalamus. Brain *41,* 619–638.

Benson, P. F. (1962) (for MacKeith, R. G.): Transient dysphagia due to muscular inco-ordination. Proc. Roy. Soc. Med. *55,* 237.

Berndt, R. S., Caramazza, A. (1980): A redefinition of the syndrome of Broca's aphasia. Appl. Psycholing. *1.3,* 221–278.

Bernstein, N. (1967): The Coordination and Regulation of Movements. Oxford: Pergamon.

Berry, M. F. (1980): Teaching Linguistically Handicapped Children. Englewood Cliffs, N. J.: Prentice-Hall.

Berry, R. J., Epstein, R., Fourcin, A. J., Freeman, M., Maccurtain, F., Noscoe, N. (1982): An objective analysis of voice disorder, Part. 1. Brit. J. Dis. Comm. *17,* 1, 67–76.

Blakeley, R. W. (1980): Screening Test for Developmental Apraxia of Speech, Tigard C. C. Publications Or.

Bloomfield, S., Marr, D. (1979): How the cerebellum may be used. Nature *227,* 1224–1228.

Blumstein, S. (1973): Some phonological implications of aphasic speech. In: Psycholinguistics and Aphasia (Goodglass, H., Blumstein, S., eds.). Baltimore: Johns Hopkins.

Blumstein, S. E., Cooper, W. E., Goodglass, H., Statlender, S., Gottleib, J. (1980): Production Deficits in Aphasia: A Voice-Onset Time Analysis. Brain and Language *9,* 153–170.

Boller, F., Albert, M., Denes, F. (1975): Palilalia. Brit. J. Dis. Comm. *10,* 92–97.

Boomer, D. S., Laver, J. (1968): Slips of the tongue. Brit. J. Dis. Comm. *3*, 2–12.

Borden, G. (1979): An interpretation of research on feedback interruption in speech. Brain and Language *7*, 307–319.

Borden, G., Harris, K. (1980): Speech Science Primer. Baltimore, Md.: Williams and Wilkins.

Boyd, I. A. (1976): The response of fast and slow nuclear bag fibres in isolated cat muscle spindles to fusimotor stimulation and the effect of the transfusal contraction on the sensory endings. Quart. J. Exp. Physiol. *61*, 203–284.

Broca, P. (1865): Sur la faculté du language articulé. Bull. Soc. Anthrop. (Paris) *6*, 337–393.

Brodal, A. (1981): Neurological Anatomy in Relation to Clinical Medicine, 3rd ed. London: Oxford University Press.

Brown, J. W. (1967): Physiology and phylogenesis of emotional expression. Brain Res. *5*, 1–14.

Brown, J. W. (1975): On the neural organisation of language. Brain and Language *2*, 18–30.

Brown, J. W. (1976): The neural organisation of language. Brain and Language *3*, 482–494.

Brunner, R. J., Kornhuber, H. H., Seemüller, E., Suger, G., Wallesch, C. W. (1982): Basal Ganglia Participation in Language Pathology. Brain and Language *16*, 281–299.

Buckingham, H. (1979): Explanation in apraxia with consequences for the concept of apraxia of speech. Brain and Language *8*, 202–226.

Byers Brown, B. (1981): Speech Therapy, Principles and Practice. Edinburgh: Churchill Livingstone.

Byrne, M. (1959): Speech and language development of athetoid and spastic children. J. Sp. Hear. Dis. *24*, 231–240.

Canning, A., Rose, M. (1974): Clinical measurement of lip and tongue movements in British children with normal speech. Brit. J. Dis. Comm. *9*, 45–50.

Canter, G. J. (1965): Speech characteristics of patients with Parkinson's disease III. J. Sp. Hear. Dis. *30*, 217–224.

Canter, G. J. (1967): Neuromotor pathologies of speech. Amer. J. Phys. Med. *46*, 659.

Critchley, E. M. R. (1981): Speech disorders of Parkinsonism: a review. J. Neurol. Neurosurg. Psychiatr. *44*, 751–758.

Crystal, D. (1981): Clinical Linguistics. (Disorders of Human Communication, Vol. 3.) Wien-New York: Springer.

Crystal, D. (1982): Terms, time and teeth. Brit. J. Dis. Comm. *17*, 3–19.

Crystal, D. (1983): Profiling Linguistic Disability. London: Edward Arnold.

Crystal, D., Fletcher, P., Garman, M. (1976): The Grammatical analysis of Language Disability. London: Edward Arnold.

Dare, M. T., Gordon, N. (1970): Clumsy children. A disorder of perception and motor organisation. Dev. Med. Ch. Neurol. *12*, 178–185.

Darley, F. L., Aronson, A. F., Brown, J. R. (1975): Motor Speech Disorders. Philadelphia-London: W. B. Saunders.

Deal, J. L., Darley, F. L. (1972): The influence of linguistic and situational variables on phonemic accuracy in apraxia of speech. J. Sp. Hear. Res. *15*, 639–653.

Denny-Brown, D. (1966): The Cerebral Control of Movement. Springfield, Ill.: Ch. C Thomas.

Dickson, D. R., Maue-Dickson, W. (1982): Anatomical and Physiological Bases of Speech. Boston: Little, Brown & Co.

Dixon, A. D. (1962): The position, incidence and origin of sensory nerve terminations in oral mucous membrane. Arch. of Oral. Biol. *7*, 39–48.

Downie, A., Low, J., Lindsay, D. (1981): Speech disorder in Parkinsonism. Usefulness of delayed auditory feedback in certain cases. Brit. J. Dis. Comm. *16*, 135–139.

Easton, T. A. (1978): Coordinative structures – the basis for a motor program. In: Psychology of Motor Behavior and Sport (Landers, D. M., Christina, R. W., eds.). Champaign IPP Human Kinetics.

Eccles, J. (1973): The Understanding of the Brain. New York: McGraw-Hill.

Edwards, M. (1973): Developmental verbal apraxia. Brit. J. Dis. Comm. *8*, 64–70.

Edwards, M. (1981): Assessment and remediation of speech. In: Advances in the Management of Cleft Palate (Edwards, M., Watson, A., eds.). Edinburgh: Churchill Livingstone.

Edwards, M. (1982): Verbal dyspraxia, a disorder of rhythm and seriation. Unpublished study.

Edwards, M., Watson, A. C. H. (eds.) (1981): Advances in the Management of Cleft Palate. Edinburgh: Churchill Livingstone.

Ellis, R., Flack, F. (eds.) (1979): Palato-glossal Malfunction. Monograph of Conference at Exeter University. London: College of Speech Therapists.

Enderby, P. (1980): Frenchay Dysarthria Assessment. Brit. J. Dis. Comm. *15*, 165–173.

Enderby, P. (1983): The Standardised Assessment of Dysarthria is possible. In: Clinical Dysarthria (Berry, W. J., ed.). San Diego, Calif.: College Hill.

Fawcus, R. (1971): Features of a psychological and physiological study of articulatory performance. Brit. J. Dis. Comm. *6*, 99–106.

Fisch, L. (1964): The function of listening and its disorders. In: Learning Problems of the Cerebrally Palsied (Loring, J., ed.). London: Spastics Soc.

Fletcher, S. (1972): Time by count measurement of diadochokinetic syllable rate. J. Sp. Hear. Res. *15*, 763–770.

Fourcin, A., Abberton, E. (1971): First applications of a new laryngograph. Med. Biol. illus. *21*, 172–182.

Fowler, C. A. (1977): Timing control in speech production. Indiana U. Lingustics Club, Bloomington. Quoted by MacNeilage, P., in: Speech Production. Language and Speech *23*, 3–22.

Franks, A. S. T. (1982): Oro-facial changes connected with normal ageing. In: Communication Changes in Elderly People (Edwards, M., ed.). London: College of Speech Therapists.

Freeman, F. J., Sands, E. S., Harris, K. S. (1978): Temporal coordination of phonation and articulation in a case of verbal apraxia. Brain and Language *6*, 106–111.

Freeman, M. A. R., Wyke, B. D. (1967): Articular Reflexes at the ankle joint. Brit. J. Surg. *54*, 990.

Freud, S. (1897): Die Infantile Cerebrallähmung. Wien: Alfred Hölder.

Fromkin, V. A. (1968): Speculations of performance models. J. Ling. *4*, 47–68.

Fromkin, V. A. (1973): Speech Errors as Linguistic Evidence. The Hague: Mouton.

Fromkin, V. A. (1980): Errors in Linguistic Performance. London-New York: Academic Press.

Gammon, S. A., Smith, P. J., Daniloff, R. G., Kim, C. W. (1971): Articulation and stress/juncture production under oral anaesthetization and masking. J. Sp. Hear. Res. *14*, 271–282.

Gazzaniga, M. S., Sperry, R. W. (1965): Language in human patients after brain bisection. Fed. Proc. *24*, 522 (abstract).

Geschwind, N. (1965): Disconnexion syndromes in animals and man. Brain *88*, 237–294, 585–644.

Geschwind, N. (1967): Discussion. In: Brain Mechanisms Underlying Speech and Language (Millikan, C. H., Darley, F. L., eds.). New York-London: Grune & Stratton.

Geschwind, N. (1975): The apraxias. Neural mechanisms of disorders of learned movement. Amer. Scientist *63*, 188–195.

Gordon, N., McKinlay, I. (1980): Helping Clumsy Children. Edinburgh: Churchill Livingstone.

Greene, M. C. L. (1980): The Voice and Its Disorders, 3rd ed. Tonbridge Wells, U.K.: Pitman Medical.

Greene, M. C. L. (1982): The Aging Voice. In: Monograph, Communication Changes in Elderly People (Edwards, M., ed.) London: College of Speech Therapists.

Greene, P. H. (1972): Problems of organisation of motor systems. In: Progress in Theoretical Biology, Vol. 2 (Rosen, R., Snell, F. M., eds.). London-New York: Academic Press.

Grewel, F. (1957): Classification of Dysarthrias. Acta Psych. et Neurol. Scand. *32*, 325–337.

Grunwell, P., Huskins, S. (1979): Intelligibility in acquired dysarthria. J. Comm. Disord. *12*, 9–22.

Gubbay, S. S. (1975): The Clumsy Child. Philadelphia-London: W. B. Saunders.

Guyette, T. W., Diedrich, W. M. (1981): A critical review of apraxia of speech. In: Speech and Language Advances in Basic Research and Practice, Vol. 6 (Lass, N. J., ed.). London-New York: Academic Press.

Guyton, A. C. (1972): Structure and Function of the Nervous System. Philadelphia-London: W. B. Saunders.

Halliday, M. A. K. (1963): The tones of English. Arch. Linguist. *15*, 1–28.

Hardcastle, W. J. (1972): The use of electropalatography in phonetic research. Phonetica *25*, 197–215.

Hardcastle, W. J. (1976): Physiology of Speech. London-New York: Academic Press.

Hardcastle, W. J., Morgan, R. A. (1982): An instrumental investigation of articulation disorders in children. Brit. J. Dis. Comm. *17*, 47–65.

Hargie, O., Saunders, C., Dickson, D. (1981): Social Skills in Interpersonal Communication. London: Croom Helm.

Hebb, D. O. (1949): The Organization of Behavior. New York: J. Wiley.

Hirose, H., Kiritani, S., Ushijima, T., Sawashima, M. (1978): Analysis of abnormal articulatory dynamics in two dysarthric patients. J. Sp. Hear. Dis. *43*, 96–105.

Hixon, T. J., Hardy, J. C. (1964): Restricted mobility of the speech articulators in cerebral palsy. J. Sp. Hear. Dis. *29*, 293–306.

Ingram, T. T. S. (1972): The classification of speech and language disorders in young children. In: The Child with Delayed Speech (Rutter, M., Martin, A., eds.). London: Heinemann Medical Books.

Irwin, O. C. (1955): Phonetic equipment of spastic and athetoid children. J. Sp. Hear. Dis. *20*, 54–57.

Israel, H. (1973): Age factor and the pattern of change in craniofacial structures. Amer. J. Phys. Anthrop. *39*, 111–128.

Itoh, M., Sasanuma, S., Ushijima, T. (1979): Velar movements during speech in a patient with apraxia of speech. Brain and Language *7*, 227–239.

Itoh, M., Sasanuma, S., Hirose, H., Yoshioka, H., Ushijima, T. (1980): Abnormal articulatory dynamics in a patient with apraxia of speech. Brain and Language *11*, 66–75.

Itoh, M., Sasanuma, S., Tatsumi, I. F., Murakami, S., Fukusako, Y., Suzuki, T. (1982): Voice-Onset time characteristics in Apraxia of Speech. Brain and Language *17*, 193–210.

Iverson, L. L. (1975): How do anti psychotic drugs work? Neurosci. Res. Prog. Bull. *13*, 29–51.

Jackson, Hughlings, J. (1968): Notes on the physiology and pathology of language. In: Selected Writings of John Hughlings Jackson (1931) (Taylor, J., ed.). London: Hodder & Stroughton. Also review in Aphasia (1935). Weisenburg, T., McBride, K. New York: Hafner.

Jakobson, R. (1968): Child Language, Aphasia and Phonological Universals. The Hague: Mouton.

Jasper, H., Ricci, G. F., Duane, B. (1960): Microelectrode analyis of cortical cell discharge during avoidance conditioning in the monkey. EEG and Clinical Neurophysiol. Suppl. 13, 139–155.

Johns, D. F. (ed.) (1978): Management of Neurogenic Communicative Disorders. Boston: Little, Brown & Co.

Johns, D. F., Darley, F. L. (1970): Phonemic variability in apraxia of speech. J. Hear. Sp. Res. *13*, 556–583.

Johns, D. F., La Pointe, L. L. (1976): Neurogenic Disorders of Output Processing: Apraxia of speech. In: Studies in Neurolinguistics, Vol. 1 (Whitaker, H., Whitaker, H. A., eds.). London-New York: Academic Press.

Jones, W. R. (1977): Electropalatography hardware. Work in progress 1. Phonetics Lab. Reading University.

Kawamura, Y. (1970): A role of oral afferents for mandibular and lingual movements. In: Oral Sensation and Perception (Bosma, J. F., ed.). Springfield, Ill.: Ch. C Thomas.

Kelso, J. A., Tuller, B. (1980): Towards a theory of apractic syndromes. Haskins Laboratories Status Report on Speech Research *SR-61*, 175–194.

Kent, R. D. (1976): Study of vocal tract characteristics in the dysarthrias. Presented to VA Workshop on Motor Speech Disorders, Madison, Wisc.

Kent, R., Netsell, R. (1975): A case study of an ataxic dysarthric: Cineradiographic and spectrographic observations. J. Sp. Hear. Dis. *40*, 115–134.

Kent, R., Netsell, R. (1978): Articulatory abnormalities in athetoid cerebral palsy. J. Sp. Hear. Dis. *43*, 353–373.

Kent, R., Netsell, R., Abbs, J. H. (1979): Acoustic characteristics of dysarthria associated with cerebellar disease. J. Sp. Hear. Res. *22*, 627–648.

Kent, R. D., Carney, P. J., Severeid, L. R. (1974): Velar movement and timing evaluation of a model for binary control. J. Sp. Hear. Res. *17*, 470–488.

Kimura, D., Archbold, Y. (1974): Motor functions of the left hemisphere. Brain 97, 337–350.

Kiritani, S., Itoh, M., Fujimura, O. (1975): Tongue pellet tracking by a computer controlled x-ray microbeam system. J. Acoust. Soc. Amer. 57, 1516–1520.

Klineberg, I. J., Greenfield, B. E., Wyke, B. D. (1970): Contributions for the reflex control of mastication from mechanoreceptors in the temperomandibular joint capsule. Dental Practit. 21, 73–83.

Koller, W. C. (1983): Dysfluency (Stuttering) in Extrapyramidal Disease. Arch Neurol. 40, 175–177.

Kornhuber, H. H. (1974): Cerebral cortex, cerebellum and basal ganglia. In: The Neurosciences, 3rd Study Program (Schmidt, F. O., Wordern, F. G., eds.). Cambridge, Mass.: MIT Press.

Kornhuber, H. H. (1977): A reconsideration of the cortical and subcortical mechanisms involved in speech and aphasia. In: Language and Hemispheric Specialisation in Man (Desmedt, J. E., ed.). Basel: Karger.

Kornhuber, H. H., Deecke, L. (1964): Hirnpotentialänderungen beim Menschen vor und nach Willkürbewegungen, dargestellt mit Magnetbandspeicherung und Rückwärtsanalyse. Arch. Ges. Physiol. Quoted by Magoun, H. W., in: Brain Mechanisms Underlying Speech and Language (Millikan, C. H., Darley, F. L., eds.). New York-London: Grune & Stratton. 1967.

Kozhevnikov, V. A., Chistovich, L. A. (1965): Speech: Articulation and Perception. Moscow: Nauka. (Transl. US Dept. of Commerce, Joint Publications Research Service, Washington.)

Kracke, I. (1975): Perception of rhythmic sequences by aphasic and deaf children. Brit. J. Dis. Comm. 10, 43–51.

Kreul, E. J. (1972): Neuromuscular control examination for parkinsonism. J. Sp. Hear. Res. 15, 72–83.

Landt, H. (1975): Oral recognition of forms and oral muscular coordination ability in dentulous subjects of various ages. Proceedings Store Kro Conference, Ascot, U.K.

La Pointe, L., Horner, J., Johns, D. F. (1975): Some phonemic characteristics in apraxia of speech. J. Comm. Dis. 8, 259–269.

La Pointe, L., Horner, J. (1981): Palilalia; a descriptive study of pathological reiterative utterances. J. Sp. Hear. Dis. 46, 34–38.

Larson, C. R., Sutton, D., Lindemann, R. C. (1978): Cerebellar regulation of phonation in rhesus monkey. Exp. Brain Res. 33, 1–18.

Lashley, K. S. (1951): The problem of serial order in behavior. In: Cerebral Mechanisms in Behavior (Jeffress, L. A., ed.). New York: J. Wiley.

Lassen, N. A., Ingvar, D. H., Skinhøj, E. (1978): Brain function and blood flow. Scient. American 239, 50–59.

Laver, J. (1970): The Production of Speech. In: New Horizons in Lingustics (Lyons, J., ed.). London: Pelican.

Laver, J. (1973): The detection and correction of slips of the tongue. In: Speech Errors as Lingustic Evidence (Fromkins, V., ed.). The Hague: Mouton.

Laver, J. (1977): Neurolinguistic Aspects of speech production. In: Grundbegriffe und Hauptströmungen der Linguistik (Gutnecht, C., ed.). Hamburg: Hoffmann und Campe.

Laver, J. (1980a): Neurolinguistic control of speech production. In: Errors in Linguistic Performance (Fromkin, V. A., ed.). London-New York: Academic Press.

Laver, J. (1980b): The Phonetic Description of Voice Quality. Cambridge: University Press.

Leanderson, R., Myerson, B. A., Persson, A. (1971): Effect of L Dopa on speech in Parkinsonism. J. Neurol. Neurosurg. Psychiat. 34, 679–681.

Lebrun, Y., Buyssens, E., Henneaux, J. (1973): Phonetic aspects of anarthria. Cortex 9, 126–135.

Lecours, A. R. (1975): Methods for the description of Aphasic Transformations of Language. In: Foundations of Language Development (Lenneberg, E. H., Lenneberg, E., eds.) New York: Academic Press.

Lecours, A. R., Rouillon, F. (1976): Neurolinguistic analysis of Jargon Aphasia. In: Studies in Neurolinguistics, Vol. 2 (Whitaker, H., Whitaker, H. A. eds.). New York: Academic Press.

Lee, J. (1980): The association between rhythmic ability and language ability. In: Language Disability in Children (Jones, F. M., ed.). Lancaster, U.K.: MTP Press.

Lencione, R. (1966): Speech and language problems in cerebral palsy. In: Cerebral Palsy (Cruikshank, W., Ralls, G., eds.). New York: Syracuse Univ. Press.

Lencione, R. (1968): A rationale for speech and language evaluation in cerebral palsy. Brit. J. Dis. Comm. *3*, 161–170.

Lenneberg, E. H. (1967): Biological Foundations of Language. New York: J. Wiley.

Lesser, R. (1978): Linguistic Investigations of Aphasia. London: Edward Arnold.

Liberman, A. M., Cooper, F. S., Harris, K. S., MacNeilage, P. F., Studdert-Kennedy, M. (1964): Some observations on a model of speech perception. In: Models for the Perception of Speech and Visual Form (Wathen-Dunn, W., ed.). Cambridge, Mass.: MIT Press.

Liepmann, H. (1900): Das Krankheitsbild der Apraxie (motorischen Asymbolie). Mschr. Psychiatr. Neurol. *8*, 15–40, 102–132, 181–197.

Logemann, J., Fisher, H. (1981): Vocal tract control in Parkinson's disease. J. Sp. Hear. Dis. *46*, 348–352.

Love, R. J., Hagerman, E. L., Taimi, E. G. (1980): Speech performance, dysphagia and oral reflexes in cerebral palsy. J. Sp. Hear. Dis. *45*, 59–75.

Luchsinger, R., Arnold, G. E. (1965): Voice, Speech and Language. London: Constable.

Luria, A. R. (1970): Traumatic Aphasia. The Hague: Mouton.

Luria, A. R. (1976): Basic Problems of Neurolinguistics. The Hague: Mouton.

Macaluso-Haynes, S. (1978): Developmental Apraxia of Speech. In: Clinical Management of Neurogenic Speech Disorders (Johns, D. F., ed.). Boston: Little, Brown & Co.

Macdonald, E. T., Aungst, L. F. (1970): Apparent independence of oral sensory functions and articulatory proficiency. In: Oral Sensation and Perception (Bosma, J., ed.). Springfield, Ill.: Ch. C Thomas.

Mackenzie, C. (1982): Aphasic articulatory defect and aphasic phonological defect. Brit. J. Dis. Comm. *17*, 27–46.

MacNeilage, P. F. (1970): Motor control of serial ordering of speech. Psychol. Review *77*, 182–196.

Magoun, H. W. (1967): Discussion. In: Brain Mechanisms Underlying Speech and Language (Millikan, C. H., Darley, F. L., eds.). New York-London: Grune & Stratton.

Martin, A. D. (1974): Some objections to the term apraxia of speech. J. Sp. Hear. Dis. *39*, 53–64.

Martin, A. D., Rigrodsky, S. (1974): An investigation of phonological impairment in Aphasia. Cortex *10*, 317–328.

Martin, J. A. M. (1981): Voice, Speech and Language in the Child. (Disorders of Human Communication, Vol. 4.) Wien-New York: Springer.

Martin, J. C. (1972): Rhythmic (hierarchical) structure versus serial structure in speech and other behavior. Psychol. Review *79*, 487–509.

Millac, P., Hassan, I., Espir, M. L. E., Slyfield, D. G. (1970): Amantadine in Parkinson's Disease. Lancet *1*, 464.

Miller, J., Hardy, W. (1962): Considerations in evaluating dysarthria. ASHA *4*, 407.

Milner, P. M. (1970): Physiological Psychology. London: Holt Rinehart & Winston.

Monrad Krohn, G. H. (1939): On facial dissociation. Act. Psychiat. *14*, 557–566.

Morley, M. (1972): Development and Disorders of Speech in Childhood, 3rd ed. Edinburgh: Churchill Livingstone.

Mountcastle, V. B. (ed.) (1980): Medical Physiology, 14th ed. St. Louis: Mosby.

Myers, R. E. (1967): Cerebral connectionism and brain function. In: Brain Mechanisms Underlying Speech and Language (Millikan, C. H., Darley, F. L., eds.). New York-London: Grune & Stratton.

Nakano, K., Zubick, H., Tyler, H. R. (1973): Speech defects of Parkinson patients. Neurol. *23*, 865–870.

Neilson, P., O'Dwyer, N. (1981): Pathophysiology of dysarthria in cerebral palsy. J. Neurol. Neurosurg. Psychiat. *44*, 1013–1019.

Netsell, R. (1971): A developing framework for research and speech production. Progress Report 1, Madison Univ., Wisc.

Netsell, R., Daniel, B., Celesia, G. C. (1975): Acceleration and weakness in Parkinsonian dysarthria. J. Sp. Hear. Dis. *40*, 170–178.

Netsell, R., Kent, R. (1976): Paroxysmal ataxic dysarthria. J. Sp. Hear. Dis. *41*, 93–109.

Netsell, R., Daniel, B. (1979): Dysarthria in adults. Arch. Phys. Med. Rehab. *60*, 502–508.

Nooteboom, S. G. (1981): Monitoring systems in the neurolinguistic control of speech production. In: Errors in Linguistic Performance (Fromkin, V., ed.). London-New York: Academic Press.

O'Dwyer, N., Quinn, P., Guitar, B., Andrews, G., Neilson, P. (1981): Procedures for verification of electrode placement in EMG studies of orofacial and mandibular muscles. J. Sp. Hear. Res. 24, 273–288.

O'Neill, Y. V. (1980): Speech and Speech Disorders in Western Thought Before 1600. Westport, Conn.: Greenwood Press.

Peacher, W. (1950): The etiology and differential diagnosis of dysarthria. J. Sp. Hear. Dis. 15, 252–265.

Penfield, W., Roberts, L. (1959): Speech and Brain Mechanisms. Princeton, N.J.: Princeton University Press.

Platt, L., Andrews, G., Howie, P. (1980): Dysarthria of adult cerebral palsy I. J. Sp. Hear, Res. 23, 28–40.

Platt, L., Andrews, G., Young, M., Quinn, P. (1980): Dysarthria of cerebral palsy 2. J. Sp. Hear. Res. 23, 41–55.

Portnoy, R. A. (1979): Hyperkinetic dysarthria as an indication of impending dyskinesia. J. Sp. Hear. Dis. 44, 214–219.

Potter, J. (1980): What was the matter with Dr. Spooner? In: Errors in Linguistic Performance (Fromkin, V., ed.). London-New York: Academic Press.

Rhines, R., Magoun, H. W. (1946): Brain Stem facilitation of cortical motor response. J. Neurophysiol. 9, 219–229.

Robertson, S. J. (1982): Dysarthria Profile. NHCSS, 59 Portland Place, London, W1.

Robinson, C. M. (1977): Rhythmic organization in speech processing. J. Exp. Psychol. Hum. Percept. 3, 83–91.

Rockey, D. (1980): Speech Disorder in 19th Century Britain. London: Croom Helm.

Rosenbek, J. C. (1978): Treating Apraxia of Speech. In: Clinical Management of Neurogenic Speech Disorders (Johns, D. F., ed.). Boston: Little, Brown & Co.

Rosenbek, J., Wertz, R. T., Darley, F. L. (1973): Oral sensation and perception in apraxia of speech and aphasia. J. Sp. Hear. Res. 16, 22–36.

Rosenbek, J., Wertz, R. T. (1976): Quoted by Wertz, Neuropathologies of speech and language. In: Clinical Management of Neurogenic Communicative Disorders. Boston: Little, Brown & Co. 1978.

Rosenbek, J., La Pointe, L. (1978): The dysarthrias. In: Clinical Management of Neurogenic Communicative Disorders (Johns, D. F., ed.). Boston: Little, Brown & Co.

Ryan, W. J. (1972): Acoustic aspects of the aging voice. Journ. of Gerontol. 27, 265–268.

Ryan, W., Burk, K. (1974): Perceptual and acoustic correlates of aging in the speech of males. J. Comm. Dis. 7, 181–192.

Samra, K., Riklan, M., Levita, E., Zimmerman, J., Waltz, J., Cooper, I. (1969): Language and speech correlates of anatomically verified lesions in thalamic surgery for Parkinsonism. J. Sp. Hear. Res. 12, 510–540.

Semmes, J. (1968): Hemispheric specialization. A possible clue to mechanism. Neuropsychol. 6, 11–26.

Shattuck-Hufnagel, S. (1979): Speech errors as evidence for a serial ordering mechanism in sentence production. In: Sentence Processing: Psycholinguistic Studies Presented to Merrill Garrett (Cooper, W. H., Walker, E. C. T., eds.). Hillsdale, N.J.: Lawrence Erlbaum Assoc.

Sparks, R. W., Helm, N., Albert, M. (1974): Aphasia rehabilitation resulting from melodic intonation therapy. Cortex 10, 303–314.

Sparks, R. W., Holland, A. L. (1976): Melodic intonation therapy for aphasia. J. Sp. Hear. Dis. 41, 287–297.

Stelmach, G. E., Diggles, V. A. (1982): Control theories in motor behavior. Acta Psychol. 50, 83–105.

Sussman, H. W. (1972): What the tongue tells the brain. Psychol. Bull. 77, 262–272.

Trost, J., Canter, C. (1974): Apraxia of speech in patients with Broca's aphasia. Brain and Language 1, 63–80.

Turvey, M., Shaw, R., Mace, W. (1979): Issues in the theory of action. In: Attention and Performance (Requin, J., ed.). Hillsdale, N.J.: Lawrence Erlbaum Assoc.

Walter Grey, W. G. (1967): Discussion. In: Brain Mechanisms Underlying Speech and Language (Millikan, C. H., Darley, F. L., eds.), pp. 190–198. New York-London: Grune & Stratton.

Walton, J. N., Ellis, E., Court, S. D. M. (1962): Clumsy children, developmental apraxia and agnosia. Brain 85, 603–612.

Welford, A. T. (1979): Principles of motor control and their application to dental problems. In: Oral Motor Behavior. National Institute of Health, N. Y.: U.S. Dept. Health Education and Welfare Workshop Proceedings.

Wertz, R. T. (1978): Neuropathologies of speech and language. In: Clinical Management of Neurogenic Communicative Disorders (Johns, D. F., ed.). Boston: Little, Brown & Co.

Whitaker, H. A. (1971): On the Representation of Language in the Human Brain. Linguistic Research Inc. Edmonton Chapmain.

Wickelgren, W. A. (1969): Context-sensitive coding, associative memory and serial ordering in (speech) behavior. Psychol. Review 76, 1–15.

Wiener, N. (1948): Cybernetics or Control and Communication in the Animals and in the Machine. New York: J. Wiley.

Williams, R., Ingham, R., Rosenthal, J. (1981): A further analysis for developmental apraxia of speech in children with defective articulation. J. Sp. Hear. Res. 24, 496–505.

Wood, F. (1980): Theoretical, methodological and statistical implications of the inhalation and CBF Technique for the study of brain and behavior relationships. Brain and Language 9, 1–8.

Wood, G. (1971): Terminology and Nomenclature. In: Handbook of Speech Pathology (Travis, L. E., ed.). New York: Appleton.

Woods, B. T., Carey, S. (1979): Language deficits after apparent clinical recovery from childhood aphasia. Ann. Neurol. 6, 405–409.

Worster Drought, C. (1974): Supra Bulbar Paresis. Spastics Int. Med. Pub. London: Heinemann Medical Books.

Wyke, B. D. (1967): The neurology of joints. Ann. Roy. Coll. Surg. Eng. 41, 25–550.

Wyke, B. D. (1970): Neurological Mechanisms in Stammering an hypothesis. Brit. J. Dis. Comm. 5, 5–15.

Wyke, B. D. (1974): Laryngeal myotatic reflexes. Fol. Phoniatr. 26, 249–264.

Yorkston, K., Beukelman, D. (1981): Assessment of Intelligibility of Dysarthric speech. C. C. Publications Tigard, Or.

Yoss, K. A., Darley, F. L. (1974): Developmental apraxia of speech in children with defective articulation. J. Sp. Hear. Res. 17, 399–416.

Zaidel, E. (1978a): Lexical organization in the right hemisphere. In: Cerebral correlates of Conscious Experience (Rougeul-Buser, A., Buser, A., eds.). Amsterdam: Elsevier.

Zaidel, E. (1978a): Lexical organization in the right hemisphere. In: Cerebral Correlates of Conscious Experience (Rougeul-Buser, A., Buser, A., eds.). Amsterdam: Elsevier.

Zemlin, W. R. (1968): Speech and Hearing Science: Anatomy and Physiology. Englewood Cliffs, N. J.: Prentice-Hall.

Author Index

Subject Index

Disorders of Human Communication

Edited by
Godfrey E. Arnold, Fritz Winckel, Barry D. Wyke

Executive Editor
Barry D. Wyke

Volume 1
Hearing: Its Function and Dysfunction
By **Earl D. Schubert**
1980. 86 figures. X, 184 pages.
ISBN 3-211-81579-1

Volume 2
Clinical Aspects of Dysphasia
By **Martin L. Albert, Harold Goodglass, Nancy A. Helm, Alan B. Rubens, and Michael P. Alexander**
1981. 12 figures. XI, 194 pages.
ISBN 3-211-81617-8

Volume 3
Clinical Linguistics
By **David Crystal**
1981. 3 figures. XII, 228 pages.
ISBN 3-211-81622-4

Volume 4
Voice, Speech, and Language in the Child: Development and Disorder
By **John A. M. Martin**
1981. 43 figures. XVI, 210 pages.
ISBN 3-211-81629-1

Volume 5
Clinical Examination of Voice
By **Minoru Hirano**
1981. 36 figures. XI, 100 pages.
ISBN 3-211-81659-3

Volume 6
Dynamics of the Singing Voice
By **Meribeth A. Bunch**
1982. 69 figures. XV, 156 pages.
ISBN 3-211-81667-4

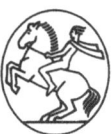

Springer-Verlag Wien New York